Why Did No One TELL ME THIS?

Running Press
Hachette Book Group
1290 Avenue of the Americas, New York, NY 10104
www.runningpress.com
@Running_Press

Printed in China

First Edition: April 2020

Published by Running Press, an imprint of Perseus Books, LLC, a subsidiary of Hachette Book Group, Inc. The Running Press name and logo is a trademark of the Hachette Book Group.

The Hachette Speakers Bureau provides a wide range of authors for speaking events. To find out more, go to www.hachettespeakersbureau.com or call (866) 376-6591.

The publisher is not responsible for websites (or their content) that are not owned by the publisher.

Interior and cover illustrations by Louise Reimer.
Print book cover and interior design by Susan Van Horn.

Library of Congress Control Number: 2019953017

ISBNs: 978-0-7624-9566-5 (paperback), 978-0-7624-9567-2 (ebook)

1010

10 9 8 7 6 5

Why Did No One TELL ME THIS?

THE DOULAS' HONEST GUIDE FOR EXPECTANT PARENTS

by **NATALIA HAILES** and **ASH SPIVAK**

illustrations by **LOUISE REIMER**

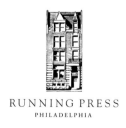

RUNNING PRESS
PHILADELPHIA

Dedicated to our moms.
And their moms, and their moms,
and their moms . . .

Contents

PART 3

PART 4

HELLO! START HERE.

Dear Readers,

HI! WE'RE NAT AND ASH, TWO BIRTH DOULAS WHO STARTED from the same place as most of you, knowing nothing about childbirth except for . . . cue GIF of a flailing crazy pregnant woman. So the idea of passing an actual human being through our vaginas was petrifying, to say the least.

But considering that millions of babies are born each year in the United States alone and that each and every one of us arrived here by the process of birth, it got us thinking: *Why is it that we all know so little about childbirth?* And, *why are we all so terrified if it's so common?*

So we started digging. And what we learned blew our minds: that we can just chill as our bodies grow tiny baby fingernails, that the uterus can grow to the size of a watermelon and then shrink back down to the size of a pear, that breast milk constantly changes its composition to fit the unique needs of the particular baby's health and developmental stages . . . The more we found out about the intricacies of the body's inner workings and defense mechanisms, the more enamored we became. And the more we explored and saw firsthand where all of our fear and misunderstanding around our bodies comes from (stay tuned!), the more it fueled our *need* to write this book.

The transition of pregnancy and childbirth is entirely transformational for each and every single person and partner that goes through it. But because it is so "ordinary," we often forget that it's actually *extraordinary.* It's a huge deal.

Having now supported hundreds of families through their pregnancies, births, and postpartum experiences—and Nat having done the deed herself with Ash as her doula!—we've put together this book as a culmination and curation of what we have learned along the way. This resource was created to help you build confidence in yourself so that you can let go and release into the craziness that is the perinatal journey. It's our goal to equip you with the tools and support to listen to your own unique, extraordinary power, to ask for help and set boundaries, and to not give a shit about the "shoulds," "should-nots," and "must-dos" that constantly flood pregnant people and partners.

What works for you may look very different than what works for your friend, your sister, or even your doctor or midwife. But *you* really and truly know best. Our hope is that this book helps you trust that.

With love and a muscle arm emoji,

Ash + Nat

P.S. One last thing: Throughout this book, we tried our best to include a wide range of birthing people and scenarios, but we recognize that depending on *your* circumstances, some of what is outlined in these pages might not always be an option for you. That's the thing about each of us being so unique! If you're a single parent, we see you. If you've experienced loss or trauma, we see you. If your baby is breech, we see you. If you're carrying more than one baby, we see you. If you or your baby have health factors that make you high risk, we see you. If you're giving your baby up for adoption, we see you. *You all matter.* Our hope is that even if everything here doesn't resonate with you, there will still be helpful bits and tools for you along the way.

WHAT IS A DOULA ANYWAY?

We know there's a lot of confusion about what we as doulas (pronounced do-la) do, so let us clear it up for you.

A birth doula is a *nonclinical* coach that provides emotional, advocacy, educational, and sometimes spiritual support during pregnancy, birth, and the immediate postpartum period.

Because we are actually *with* clients for so much of their labor (you won't see most clinical providers until later in your labor, and even then, if you are birthing in a hospital, you may not see them until it's time to push) and we are not bound to institutional policies, we have a unique vantage point on this process. Basically, we get access to the stuff no one else sees!

Doula support looks different for everybody, but some examples of what a doula can do include:

- Help you navigate conversations with your care provider about your pregnancy.
- Help you cope during early labor before you are with your clinical provider.
- Help you decide when to go to your birthing place during labor.
- Help you avoid unnecessary interventions.
- Help you find ways to encourage the baby to descend through the birth canal while you have an epidural.
- Provide hands-on support, like massage, during labor.
- Assist with lactation once the baby is here.
- Allow for your partner to take a break.
- Help you process your birth experience and adjust to parenthood in the postpartum period.

People often ask us if—since we've seen so much—we would still want a doula for our own births. We may be biased, but our answer is always, *"We'd take two."*

Common Myths about Doulas

A DOULA AND A MIDWIFE ARE THE SAME.

Nope! Midwives are *clinical* providers, which means that you'd use a midwife *instead* of an OBGYN. While there are different requirements per state, licensed and certified midwives have either gone through nursing school or years of clinical training. Midwives can catch babies in hospitals, birth centers, or your home. You can have a midwife *and* a doula, but they are definitely not interchangeable! See page 195 for more on the differences between midwives and OBGYNs.

DOULAS ARE FOR HOME BIRTHS ONLY OR FOR "ALL-NATURAL BIRTHS."

In our practices, 90 percent of the births we support take place in hospitals. And while we are certainly specially trained to help people achieve nonmedicated births when the labor and baby are cooperating, many of our clients come to us already certain that an epidural—or in some cases, cesarean surgery—is the right choice for them. Doulas support *you* doing *you*.

MY PARTNER IS VERY SUPPORTIVE, SO I DON'T NEED A DOULA.

Doulas don't replace your partner. In fact, our job is to make it *easier* on your partner and take some of the pressure off them. Remember, this is a very emotional time for your partner too—even if they don't show it!—and if this is their first child, they've never done this before either. Our job is to normalize the process, allow them to take a break or get a sandwich without leaving you alone, and assist with the logistics so that they can actually be a *better* partner.

DOULAS ARE A COOL ACCESSORY FOR THE RICH.

Actually, research shows that having a doula provides real benefits[1] for your birth, including:

- more likely to rate your childbirth experience positively
- less likely to need Pitocin
- less likely to have a C-section
- less likely to use pain medication
- more likely for your baby to have a higher 5-minute APGAR score (this is an initial measurement of your baby's health)

The cost of having a doula can range from nothing to thousands of dollars. Many work on a sliding scale, and sometimes you can get your insurance company or flexible spending account (FSA) to cover some or all of the money. You can also ask friends to contribute to the cost of a doula on your gift registry if you plan on having a baby shower. For those for whom cost is truly prohibitive, there are programs that offer no- and low-cost doulas, so be sure to do an online search for what is available in your area. Typically, doulas are ready to rally to support those in want and need. Just ask!

SETTING THE FOUNDATION

Our bodies are crazy smart.

Even while pregnant, your body is yours. You are the boss.

Birth is an experience, not solely an outcome.

There is no "right" way to birth. Your way is the only way.

Ask for help—lots of it.

Postpartum matters.

part

1

DROWNING OUT THE NOISE AND LEARNING TO LISTEN TO YOU

TO BEGIN, LET US FIRST SAY, HOLY SHIT, AMAZING JOB! Being pregnant isn't always easy. And though hopefully there are lots of special moments throughout, you certainly don't get enough recognition for all you have to go through to get here and be here. Dude, look what you are already doing—you're freaking growing a human! We bow down to you.

But we recognize that the perinatal period can also bring up a lot of stuff. The stakes are so high, and it touches on everyone's biggest fears: giving up control, change, loss, and the unknown. *(When's my labor going to start? How long will it last? What will it feel like? What will my baby be like? Will they have all their toes?)* All the while your hormones are going crazy, *and* you have to lug around another human everywhere you go!

So while having a baby can be wonderful, a blessing, yadda yadda yadda, it is also *very* normal to feel utterly afraid, anxious, and like, *How am I going to do this?!*

We want to invite you to approach this time as an opportunity. While this may be one of the hardest and most uncomfortable things you ever do, all this baby growing allows for some incredible personal growing along the way.

We all arrive at this transition with different experiences, histories, traumas, triumphs, circumstances, and bodies. We are each the sum of all of these things.

And our babies are the sum of their own bodies, experiences, and circumstances *in addition* to all of yours—which is why *you* are *so* equipped to help them navigate their new world!

No two people can possibly have the same *collection* of experiences. So it is actually *impossible* for your birth or your baby to be the same as anyone else's—not your sister's, or your mom's, or the woman at the grocery store's (especially hers!). And since each of our *collections* is unique, that means it's also impossible for all of those standards, musts, must-nots, and must-haves surrounding pregnancy to work perfectly for you or your baby. *You* get to filter what feels right. *You* get to create your own story. *You* get to forge your *own* path as you go along.

Our Collections

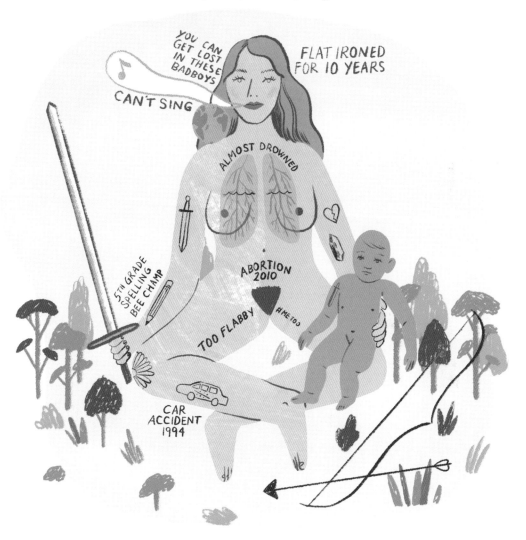

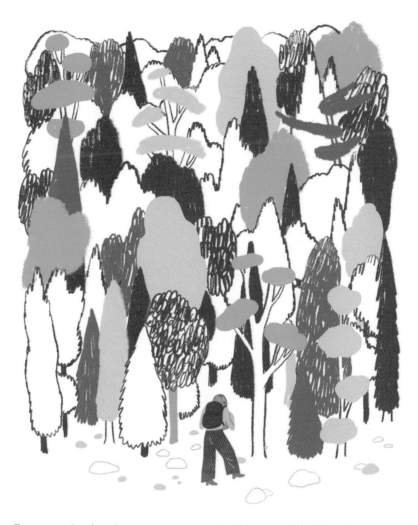

For some, this freedom is exciting and exhilarating! And for others, it can feel intimidating, overwhelming, and hard to know where to begin. Which way do you walk if there is no path laid out in front of you? How do you make it through the unknown without directions?

While we can't predict what will arise on your path, we do know that your path will likely be different from what you are imagining and it will likely be changing all the time. Focusing on the path alone seems almost silly if it's not within our

10

control and is constantly changing anyway. But what we can influence is how we move through it.

And we have a secret to share—do you want to know the best thing about not having control over the perinatal period? The pressure is off! Of course we want to *influence* as much as we can, and to set ourselves up for success, but there is actually *only so much we can do.* Sigh of relief.

So how do we not stay so focused on *"the* path"? How do we stay agile and flexible, while also valuing the need to stop and pause along the way to check in and ensure we are making decisions based on what is *actually true* for us at each moment?

So glad you asked!

We each have a compass inside to help us navigate and find our way. What do we mean by "a compass inside"? You're about to find out! This section is all about helping you *tune in* to that compass and ensuring you have the appropriate support you need throughout the process to trust it. Because you don't need to do this alone! Forging our own paths is hard. We need people to let us ugly cry when we've *had it,* make us laugh when we fall on our face, and let us pass out on their couch when we just need a damn change of scenery. And we need to make sure we have the clinical support to help us avoid unnecessary roadblocks whenever possible.

Before we dive into the specifics of pregnancy, birth, and the postpartum period, we want you to really learn to listen to your own instincts. To do that, we've put together some exercises in the following pages. You may be tempted to skip over them. We totally get it, but this is the part where we ask you to trust *us* and give them a try. While one exercise may not resonate, another may allow for a whole slew of dots to be connected for you.

And just a heads-up: You will be exploring your personal and family history here, so if at any point you feel that it is too much, stop and take a break. That's you *tuning in* to your own compass! If you sense that something big may come up for you, please wait to do the exercise with someone who can help you process what you are feeling.

TUNING IN:
LEARNING TO LISTEN TO YOU

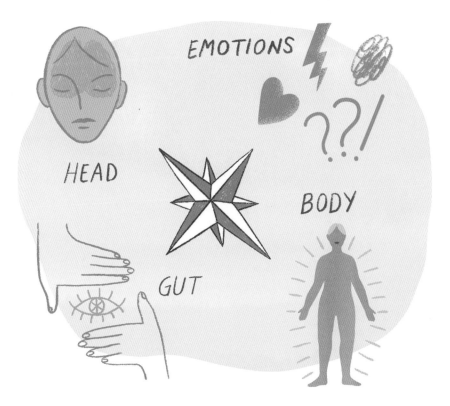

Let's begin with a framework for how you can *tune in.*

Meet the compass inside you, or your "four directions" to help you navigate your *perinatal path.* (Sorry, we couldn't help ourselves.)

It's cool if this sounds totally cheesy. It is. But it's also a *powerful* framework, so stick with us as you learn about this tool!

First things first. How do you *tune in*? Easy! You simply pause, close your eyes, breathe, and check in with each of your four navigators for guidance. (We'll walk you through those below and give you excercises in the following pages.)

12

Now, we are all very familiar with the *Head*. The Head helps us solve problems, strategize, discern, ask questions, and speak. You're using it to read this book right now! But not everything, especially during the perinatal period, can be understood or processed through the Head alone. Our Heads take in so much information each day from social media, the internet, day-to-day activities, friends, family, the stranger on the train, popular culture and can talk us into and out of just about anything—*I could do this, no I should do that, or maybe it's best to do both*—making it hard to know what is actually *true* or *real* for *us*, within the context of our unique *collections*.

With all of those factors playing together, you can see why it's nearly impossible for our most familiar pilot to cut it on its own in this terrain. That's why you have your *Body, Emotions,* and *Gut* to help. These are powerful copilots, yet so few of us have been taught to trust them as a navigation tool or have even been shown that it is safe to do so.

13

Our experiences become part of us and the *collections* that we carry. And each of these experiences, particularly the negative or traumatic ones from our childhoods as well as the acute traumas in adulthood, can "calcify" inside of us, blocking us from being able to know what we *truly* want or need—or trust that we are capable and deserving of getting it. While these *blocks* originally formed to protect us from getting hurt again, it doesn't mean they are still serving us today in their current shape or size. But these blocks *can change!* They can become smaller, lighter, or more permeable to outside influence. They can even transform into influential permanent fixtures inside of us, sprouting new parts that become fresh sources of fuel—our *power plants* that allow for brand-new possibilities.

But in order for our blocks to shift and transform, we must be able to *tune in* and find the ones that need nourishing, or at least notice where they live inside of us and get the support we need to work *with* them.

How do you start *tuning in*? How do you let your Body, Gut, and Emotions start guiding alongside your Head? The first step is simply to try!

One of the coolest aspects of the perinatal period is that you've already started doing it. And your baby is helping you! You feel when your baby kicks, which makes you more aware of your *Body* and in turn builds trust that your Body is growing those feet as you watch *Queer Eye.* You are letting your *Emotions* take over as you cry at that ridiculous commercial. And perhaps you've gone with your *Gut* and called your provider once or twice because something just felt off, or perhaps you've started to have magical feelings or dreams about your baby, noticing new synchronicities around you.

In other words: You're already using your compass!

The following pages will help you continue to build your ability to *tune in:* to remember you and baby are in this together and to help your Head be a bit less noisy so you can actually hear what your Body, Gut, and Emotions are saying. They will also help you locate where some of your blocks live, give you tools to work *with* them, and ensure you are setting yourself up with the support you need for this transition.

C'mon let's go!

LET THAT BABY GUIDE YOU

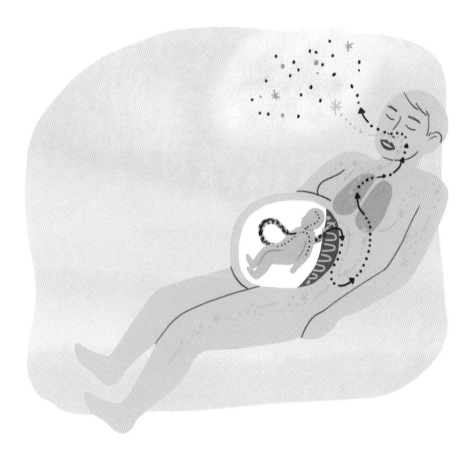

We often think it's our job as parents to show our kids the way—and it is. But they are also our biggest teachers. When we don't have the answer or aren't sure what to do, baby may actually be able to show us, if we are willing to listen. After all, babies have their own compass, and their Body, Gut, and Emotions don't have a fully developed Head to hold them back yet!

Here's an exercise that will help you continue to trust that your baby has innate wisdom for you to learn from and you guys are in this thing together—all the way!

BREATHING WITH BABY

Read this whole exercise through first, and then close your eyes and give it a go.

- Close your eyes, put your hands on your belly, and take nice, long, deep inhales and exhales. If you feel your baby move, say *Hi!*

- Focus on the sensation of the air passing through the rims of your nostrils as you breathe.

- Start to trace how the oxygen travels from your body to baby's body and back out of your body.

  - Imagine the oxygen's path. You can watch the oxygen travel as light, a color, or liquid. You can feel it move through you as heat, moisture, or a tingling sensation, or you can hear it as sound. Choose whichever resonates most for you.

- Follow the oxygen along this route:

  - It passes through the rims of your nostrils and into your throat. It is then filtered for you by your windpipe. The good stuff is passed on to your lungs, then into your bloodstream to your uterus, through the placenta and cord, and into baby's belly where it will circulate through baby's bloodstream. Then all the carbon dioxide—the stuff baby doesn't need—travels back out the cord, into the placenta, through the uterus, back into your bloodstream, to your lungs, and back out the rims of your nostrils.

- Take a few deep breaths while tracing the oxygen, and as you inhale remember that oxygen is nutrient-rich. It is exactly what is helping your baby grow and thrive. And all you need to do to help your baby grow and thrive is inhale. *You're doing it!*

- As you exhale, recognize that you are ridding both you and baby of the stuff you no longer need—your waste. The only thing you have to do for this to happen is exhale. *It's that easy!*

○ As you are breathing with your baby in this way, feel free to ask a question, send a little message, or just say *What's up?*

You can do this whenever, wherever, to tune in and connect to your body!

#BrilliantTIP

If you are someone who is anxious about your baby's well being, learning how to do kick counts can be reassuring.[2] Warning: for others, kick counts can cause unnecessary stress. So go with what feels right for you!

WHAT IS YOUR BODY TELLING YOU?!

Connecting with your baby is a great way to connect with your Body. After all, your baby kind of forces you to, ready or not, as your Body has already jumped into the driver's seat to grow that baby anyway.

We know listening to what your Body is telling you can be scary, since most of us have a zillion reasons why we have a *complicated* relationship with it. But here's the thing about the Body (and why we are starting with this point on the compass): If you can learn to trust it and feel safe in it, it can actually *help you* build up your connection to your Gut, as well as *ground you* when your Head or Emotions feel too strong or out of control.

So we need to build back up that trust so your Head feels safe letting your Body take the lead. How? Start listening and practicing! The following exercises were designed to help you do just that.

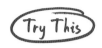

NANCY DREW-IN' IT

Throughout the day, check in with the sensations that arise in your body. (We even suggest going so far as recording them.) How do certain *places* affect those sensations? Certain vibes or the decor of a room? Certain people? The time of day? The food you eat? What are the sensations you feel when you know you are angry, sad, excited? What sensations do you feel when you like something? What goes on when you don't like something? And go the other way too—if you feel a sensation in your body first, ask yourself: *Where* are you? *Who* are you with? Can you discern *what* is causing those sensations to arise?

It's different for everybody, but here are some of the ways your Body may talk to you:

- Tingling feelings
- Warm or cold sensations
- Shivers
- Itchiness
- Tightness in chest
- Releasing fluids (blood, tears, saliva, vaginal fluids, milk)
- Nausea
- A pit in your stomach
- Needing to go to the bathroom
- Butterflies in your stomach
- Aches or pains
- Restlessness or bouncing of legs, fingers, hands
- Facial and/or eye twitches

- Tension in the jaw, shoulders, neck
- Hunger
- Bloating
- A feeling of spaciousness inside, an opening or a feeling of flowing
- Feeling very light or like you are floating
- Feeling like your body is very heavy
- Feeling stuck or frozen
- Speaking on your vocal cords (vocal fry)
- Speaking especially softly, loudly, fast, or slow
- Burning

18

Of course, some sensations will be directly related to your pregnancy (thanks, baby!), but you'll likely still be surprised by the patterns you find. Take note!

BODY BLOCKS

Now that you have an idea of the language your Body uses to talk to you, let's explore your relationship with your Body. Find a private, quiet place to do this one, and get a pen and paper ready. Read through the exercise below before you begin.

- Find a comfortable position and close your eyes. Take nice, long inhales and exhales.

- Keeping your eyes closed and breathing deeply, begin to scan your body, starting from your head and ending at your toes. To scan your body, call to mind each individual part of your physical self, both internal and external—head, jaw, shoulders, throat, lungs, uterus, stomach, cervix, legs, toes, etc.

- As you scan, take notice of what pops up for you as you address each part. Look for any colors, images, people, smells, body sensations, thoughts, or memories even if they seem irrelevant. Note any resistance and any parts you wanted to skip over.

- If you feel any resistance at certain parts or tension, see if you can use your breath to help release it by sending a long, audible exhale in the direction of the tension.

When you are done scanning, open your eyes and write down any emotions, sensations, or points of interest that came up for you. Once you've reflected on your scan, ask yourself the following questions to find your *blocks:*

- Did you have resistance to this exercise overall? Was sitting and being with your body difficult for you to do? Were you able to be still?

- Did anything surprising come up?

- Is the language you used to describe your parts, thoughts, or memories positive, negative, neutral?

- Which body parts felt strongest? What did you celebrate about yourself? Where are your *power plants*?

- How much of the language, imagery, and ideas that arose:

  - come from a place of judgment?

  - are actually true to you today?

  - are actually not about *your* body, but someone else's?

- Did anything come up that might be good to share with your birth and support team?

- Based on this information, are there ways your support team may be able to make you feel safer during the perinatal period?

DROPPING IN

Now that you have located where some of your blocks may be and are thinking about the support you may need around them, we can start practicing how to use our Bodies and *power plants* to ground ourselves when we get overwhelmed by our Heads or just a need a little break. Read this exercise all the way through first, then close your eyes.

1   Sit with both feet flat on the floor, stand, or lay flat on your back.

2   Close your eyes and put your hands on your belly.

3   Turn the edges of your lips upward very slightly, as if you were smiling. (Feel for tension in your jaw releasing as you do this.)

4   Take long, deep breaths in and out of your nose, focusing on *the sensation* of air hitting the edges of your nostrils as it comes in and out.

5   *Feel* your belly and chest rise and fall with each inhale and exhale. Challenge yourself to inhale and exhale for as long as you can—how full and how empty can you make your belly and chest?

6   Feel and listen to the rhythm of your heart beating. You can also put your hand on your chest to feel it.

7   Having trouble? Where are your *power plants*? Focus on those. Or feel for your baby if you'd like. Can you sense them moving around? Any fingers swooshing? Try not to judge *how* it feels for your baby to be inside of you. Instead just let it be an acknowledgment that they are present and a part of you that can offer help.

8   Anytime you start to feel overwhelmed again, it's okay! Simply turn the edges of your lips back upward, take a deep inhale, an audible exhale, and bring your focus back onto any of the aforementioned sensations, your *power plants*, or your baby. Don't try to escape your thoughts: it's totally cool for them to be there. Just bring your focus to your sensations instead.

9   Whenever you are ready, take a final long inhale and exhale, and open your eyes.

How'd that feel?

Get this: you can *drop in* to your Body anytime you want. You're stuck with your Body anyway, so you might as well start hanging out with it. The more you do it, the better it will start feeling, and the easier it will be to ground yourself. So just keep practicing!

GO WITH YOUR GUT: #THISISHOWIWASBORN

As you start building your relationship back up with your Body, you are automatically building up a connection with your Gut too. Often, the Gut speaks to us via the Body. It is because of the Gut—aka our instincts, or the things that come to us that we *know* are real and true without fully knowing *why* or *how*—that we have survived as a species. The Gut is what reminds us that we are connected to everyone that came before us, through our baby, our own birth, and our Body! And though we try to cover up our animalistic ways by wearing nice clothes and using a microwave, we are definitely still animals—which means, we have awesome instincts!

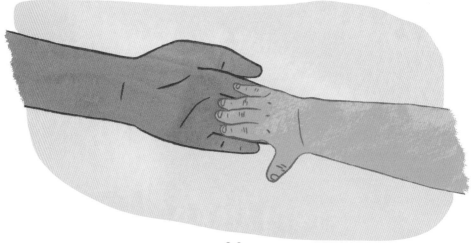

What follows is a conversation guide to help you learn more about how you got here, based around the experience of your own birth. This exercise is meant to help you remember that you are not in this alone and that birth is what connects you to a very, very long line of birthers before you. Use this tool to keep the conversation going with your Gut when your Head makes it hard to hear.

But first, a quick disclaimer: Keep in mind, *how* you got here is *not* a reflection of how your baby will get here. So please don't let this exercise set any expectations for your experience or use it as a point of comparison later on. If you can't or don't want to talk with the person who birthed you, skip to the next part.

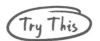

A CONVERSATION GUIDE

Seek out the person who birthed you and ask:

- Where was I born?

- Who was there?

- How did you know you were in labor?

- How do you remember the experience overall?

- What was most enjoyable about it?

- What was most difficult?

- Did you feel supported? What made you feel supported? What made you feel unsupported?

- Were medications used? What was that like?

- Was I born via C-section? If so, how come? What was that like? How did you feel about it?

- Were there any complications?

- Did I have to go to the neonatal intensive care unit? If so, why?

- What was your transition into parenthood like?

- Did I breast/chest-feed? If so, how soon after being born? And for how long overall? What was that experience like?

- What was your postpartum experience like?

- Did you have support postpartum? What was most helpful? What type of support did you wish you had that you didn't?

For those who don't or can't have access to the person who birthed you, feel that this exercise is inappropriate, or just don't want to go there, remember that you are still connected to the history of birth. You come from a long line of birthers and how *you* got here *is not* a reflection of what is to come. *You get to create a whole new story.*

Here are a few questions you can ask others and yourself:

- For those who want to, ask adoptive parents, relatives, or anyone else you wish to connect with about any details they may have about your birth and/or what it was like to meet you for the first time.

- Are there any people in your life you think are freakin' awesome and have given birth before? Can you ask them what their experience giving birth was like? Use the questions above to guide the conversation if you want!

- Are there any historical or spiritual figures, people, or characters that you draw strength from?

Don't forget to share anything you think will be helpful with your support team!

YOUR EMOTIONS ARE TELLING YOU IMPORTANT SHIT

Sometimes, our Emotions and feelings are easy to access—so much so that it can feel like we are drowning in them. Other times, our emotions are harder and more confusing to understand, or we don't think they are worthy of our time and energy because we're *doing just fine*.

But our Emotions and feelings are always true.

And *lots* of Emotions can come up in the perinatal period.

24

Here is a way for you to start breaking down your Emotions and get the information you need from them.

Note: If at any point you feel like your Emotions are too much, remember you can *drop in* to your Body. We also want to acknowledge that PMAD—perinatal mood and anxiety disorders—are real. And they aren't always extreme. Sometimes they can show up as depression, or anxiety, or both. So even if what you are experiencing doesn't seem so severe, having dedicated emotional support during this huge transition can be game changing. See pg 201 for more.

READING YOUR EMOTIONS

Step One

Name your Emotion (here are a few ideas to get you started):

○ Guilt	○ Love	○ Resentment	○ Confusion
○ Shame	○ Frustration	○ Worry	○ Stress
○ Excitement	○ Anger	○ Anxiety	○ Tired
○ Fear	○ Sadness	○ Boredom	○ Apathy
○ Jealousy	○ Joy	○ Hate	

Are you unsure of what you are feeling? Our Emotions often speak to us through the Body. So *Nancy Drew* it. What sensations do you feel or not feel? Are there certain sensations familiar to you that are indicators of certain feelings? Your baby may even have some feedback for you!

Step Two

Why am I feeling this way?

- o Is this emotion fresh or is it resurfacing from something in the past?

- o Do I feel seen or heard?

- o Do I feel safe?

- o Do I feel worthy?

- o Do I feel loved or supported?

- o Did I cross someone else's boundary?

- o Did someone else cross my boundary?

- o Was there a loss?

- o Is it actually just not affecting me/that big of a deal?

- o Am I in the middle of a transition or change (this includes your pregnancy!)?

- o What's happening with my hormones? (A lot in pregnancy!)

- o Are someone else's emotions making me feel a certain way?

- o Do I feel judged?

- o Am I trying to look a certain way or be something for someone else's standards or expectations?

- o Where am I physically when I feel this way?

- o Who am I with when I feel this way?

- o Do I need to forgive myself or someone else?

- o Is there something I can take responsibility for?

- o Is there something I don't want to confront?

- o Is there something I don't have control over?

If you have found the real root or truth behind your emotion, your Body will often respond. You may experience a release—your muscles might relax, you might cry, shake, laugh, scream in anger—or you may suddenly feel lighter. Or, you may experience a contraction—your shoulders tense, your Body's posture changes so that you're physically smaller or more compact, your breathing gets quicker. Take note—in both scenarios, your Body is telling you that you've hit on gold! You are starting to work with your Emotions. If your Body isn't giving you feedback or the Emotion feels stuck or won't go away, it is possible that you haven't gotten to the real, honest, root cause of it yet, or it may simply not be the right time or place to address it. And that's okay! It will happen when you are ready. Professional support may be helpful.

Step Three

If you experienced a release, it may be that coming to terms with the honest why behind your Emotion was enough to move it through you and not let it get stuck. You may have even transformed a *block*!

If you experienced a contraction, it may be that you are hitting on one of those more difficult *blocks*. We mention this because it is possible for some of these bigger *blocks* to unexpectedly surface during the perinatal period. Maybe you already know the wheres and whys of some of these, or maybe you don't yet. Maybe you feel ready to start transforming them, or maybe they still feel protective in their current shape.

It's all good! What we hope you can walk away with is the understanding that all Emotions are true—you are not silly or stupid for feeling whatever it is you are feeling. And all Emotions have really powerful energy behind them. So, if we can nurture our *blocks* instead of shying away from them, we can then harness the energy behind our Emotions and put their power toward what we want to create. Our Emotions can be the force behind some pretty powerful shit!

Here's how you can start nurturing your blocks:

- Feel all the feels: Cry, scream, snuggle, roar, bubble over with joy, laugh!

- Take an action to repair something that was broken or needs to be fixed.

- Communicate what needs to be communicated.

- Self-care routines and rituals.

- Restate or reestablish a boundary.

- Change the language of your personal monologue. (See below.)

- Take an action that can bring you closer to effecting change.

- Forgive yourself or others.

- Take responsibility.

- Get support!

THE SOUNDTRACK IN YOUR HEAD

We saved the Head for last because we wanted you to first have the tools to communicate with your Body, Gut, and Emotions so that you can use them to help you sort through that *personal soundtrack* of yours—you know, the thing that yaps at you all day long, going through the to-do lists over and over again, judging, discerning, wandering elsewhere during boring conversations, absorbing the world around you, and making it hard to know what is actually true amid all that noise.

The goal here isn't to get *rid* of the soundtrack. Instead, we want to become more *aware* of it—the language we use to talk to ourselves, which characters play the biggest roles, which story lines are on repeat, and where we go in our fantasies

. . . because when we stop to listen, our Head is actually giving us a lot of valuable information about some deep-seated fears, true desires, and our overall relationship to our selves.

By *examining* our thoughts in this way, by *questioning* them, instead of immediately *absorbing them as fact,* we can start using our Body, Gut, and Emotions to put our Heads at ease when they are being unreasonable. We can start locating some of our *blocks*. And, we can actually start *using* our Heads to nurture those *blocks* so that they can start sprouting new parts for us to derive energy and fuel from (our *power plants!*), instead of having them drain us.

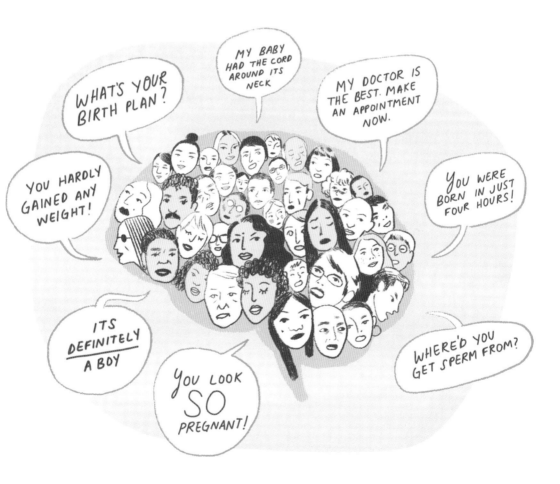

We are going to lead you through another exercise. Try not to judge or edit yourself here. The gold is in seeing what's actually going on inside your Head. We know that getting to know yourself on this level can be scary, but your personal soundtrack is *not* a reflection of who you are. Instead, you can think of it as a collection of ideas that were passed down to you, passed off on you, or patterned in you. So get it all out on paper. The more we can recognize the patterns and language living up in there, the closer we can get to freeing ourselves of them—or at least not having them be so loud!

EXPLORING YOUR PERSONAL SOUNDTRACK

Part One

- Get a pen and paper.

- Make a list of what's keeping you up at night—other than your bladder. Try to leave some space between each thought, as there will be follow-up questions for each.

  - Start with the to-do lists that are crowding your headspace—work-related, family-related, baby-related, etc. *"I should have gotten a crib by now."*

  - Now go deeper: what is stressing you out? *"My partner has been coming home late every night." "My big deadline at work is on Tuesday."*

  - And now dig really deep and write down the big fears, anxieties, and what-ifs that keep coming up. *"My vagina will never work again after birth." "What if I lose the baby?"*

If you feel stuck or aren't sure, time two minutes on your phone, close your eyes, take a few deep inhales and exhales, and brain dump everything you hear yourself think on that piece of paper.

Part Two

- ○ Read your list.

- ○ What words or phrases do you see yourself repeating? Maybe some *what-ifs, need-tos, won'ts, shoulds, can'ts,* or *not-enoughs*? Perhaps some *lates* or *nevers*? Is there an overall tone or energy you are picking up on? Is there a specific person or people that keep showing up? Circle the patterns that you find, and/or mark the tone/energy of your voice. This is the language that you use to talk to yourself *all day long!* Make a note of that, and we'll come back to this soon.

- ○ Now, use your Body, Gut, and Emotions to check in with each thought and see, *Is this actually mine? Is it true?*

  - **Your Body:** What sensations do you feel, or not feel? See pg 18 for help.

  - **Your Gut:** Whose voice do you hear? Is someone else speaking it to you—like your mom, a sister, a friend, or a character on TV? If you are visualizing it, *who* is it happening to? Are you actually there or are you *watching* a scenario? Is it you as an adult or you as a child?

  - **Your Emotions:** What Emotions come up? Why do you think you are feeling that way? See pg 25 for help.

- ○ Put a big *X* next to the thoughts/fears that you realize aren't yours or don't actually feel true to you *today*—all the thoughts/worries you realize you are *watching,* are in someone else's voice, were true for a younger version of yourself, cause your body to maintain a neutral reaction, or just don't really resonate or cause strong emotions to percolate. Take that in for a moment. That's huge! And very helpful to remember.

◉ For the thoughts/worries still left—the ones that really do feel true ask yourself the following questions and write the answers down next to the thought/worry.

1. *Are there any actions I can take to make myself feel safer or more secure around this particular thing?* For example, could you get extra postpartum support, some self-care, talk to your practitioner, or mark on your calendar a deadline to purchase an item?

2. *Is a boundary being broken or encroached on?* If the answer is yes, what steps can you take to reset or define that boundary with others, or reestablish it for yourself? For example, if the thought had to do with your partner never being home, is there a conversation to be had where new requests are made? If the thought had to do with too many people visiting you postpartum, can you set up a visiting schedule ahead of time so people have expectations of when and for how long they will be staying?

3. *Why is this person manspreading in my Head?* Are you comparing yourself to them? Do they make you feel loved and safe? Do they make you feel nervous or like you need to impress them? Are you worried about how they feel about you? Do you miss them? Is there an action you can take, something you can communicate, or some self-care you can do so they take up less space in there?

4. *Is this something that I actually have control over?* If the answer is no, let that sit with you for a second. If you can't control it anyway, is it worth your energy? Is there a phrase or mantra that can help you remember this? Perhaps, *"I trust it will work out."*

5. *Is this something I need to worry about today?* Do you have time before you need to deal with this thing? Can you return to this worry at a later date? For example, do you really need to worry about a pumping schedule for going back to work today? Do you want to mark on your calendar a time that *would be* appropriate to think about this thing again so that you don't forget? (Seriously. Whip out the calendar!)

Part Three

- Get a fresh piece of paper and write up top: "I am committing to . . ."

- Look back over the phrases you've circled in the beginning and pick a particular phrase, pattern, word, tone, or story that you see repeating itself. Now change it.

   For example, maybe all of your *can'ts* become *"I will figure out hows."* Or your *"I shoulds"* become *"I trust that I'll get done what actually needs to get done."* And your *"I was never good at sports, how am I going to birth my baby?"* becomes *"I work twelve-hour shifts; my body knows how to work hard!"* You get the idea.

- Pick one thought you commit to working on changing and write it down on this new piece of paper.

- Read back through your answers to the questions above. Pick 1–3 action items that feel doable and implementable. If you are someone who tends to overcommit, start with just one.

- Write down what you are committing to on this page and mark that calendar where appropriate. (Really!)

For the next two weeks, your priority is whatever you have written on this page. Take those actions. Reestablish those boundaries. Continuously check in with your personal soundtrack—you don't need to redo this whole exercise, just pause and listen to what's happening up in there throughout the day—so that you can replace the language with which you talk to yourself.

This is a *huge* first step in starting to change the shape of those *blocks*. But it can take time, so be patient with yourself! You will likely still get frustrated and anxious during this time. The first step is just noticing this. Keep these lists and return to them whenever you feel ready to commit or recommit to the coping tools you have created for yourself.

GETTING SUPPORT: SETTING THE RECORD STRAIGHT (WTF?!)

Now that you have flexed your *tuning in* skills, let's talk about support. We've already had you take note of where and how support may be useful. So now let's focus on *who* can help you move through the perinatal period with more ease—because it's not all on you! We'll help you build your squad.

We're going to begin with your clinical care. While the rest of your squad is key, your clinical care will make the biggest difference to your actual birth experience and transition into parenthood. And we want to make sure you are setting yourself up to have the clinical support that can *actually* support you. Because just as our culture has made our abilities to *tune in* more difficult, it has also had some major implications on our reproductive health care system.

We're about to share some not-so-fun stats. Bear with us—this is important.

Today, the United States has the worst maternal mortality rates among developed nations—with best estimates saying *half* could be avoided.[3] Black women* are four times more likely than white women* to die in childbirth, regardless of any other factors,[4] and one-third of women* *report* having birth trauma,[5] meaning the actual number is likely higher. Yet we spend *way more* money on maternal care than other nations that have better outcomes.[6]

So what is going on? In emergency situations, birth in the United States has come *such* a long way, and it certainly isn't that our clinical providers don't *want* to provide excellent care.

When we asked ourselves this question, we realized that we needed to travel back in time to understand. And we learned that the story really begins with the birth of our country. There's actually a pretty clear through line we can follow that shows us how we ended up where we are today.

*language used in studies and sources

Some of the History We Can't Ignore

Let's start at the birth of our nation. In colonial America, white women were led to believe that they were facing eternal judgment from God based on how they birthed (#nopressure). Many coping techniques utilized by midwives were considered "magic" and therefore banned, and it was considered indecent for white women to make too much noise while in labor (#helpful). Meanwhile, black women and their babies were considered to be the property of someone else. What a foundation to build on!

During the mid-nineteenth century, the white elite were largely replacing female midwives with male physicians coming back from training in Europe. But this was not because the way of the physician was more advanced, or because midwifery did not work. In fact, as childbirth historian Irvine Loudon says, "If I was forced to identify one factor above all others as the determinant of high maternal mortality in the USA, I would unhesitatingly choose the standard of the obstetric training in the medical schools; not only the content but also the attitudes instilled by these schools."[7]

Physicians proliferated because of high-powered consumer demand; in white colonial America, working with one became a sign of status. It was much more difficult for women to become formally educated, and even more difficult for women of color (though some beat the odds—Google Rebecca Lee Crumpler), so midwives couldn't go to school or organize. And without funds, education, and the ability to organize, midwives had no way to compete.

These first physicians were trained to use forceps as the standard of care, even though the misapplication of forceps resulted in increased perineal lacerations, uterine trauma, and fetal defects in patients.[8] But these doctors were charging money, so they had to justify their worth by doing something. For the first time ever, the rich were more likely to die during childbirth than the poor—because the poor were working with midwives instead of "fancy" physicians.[9]

Medical misinformation flourished during this time. Outlandish claims by medical journals included the idea that black women didn't feel pain[10], white women were incapable of giving birth without their doctors rescuing them, and

35

birth pain would be the worst agonies known to them, greater than what soldiers experienced during the Civil War.[11] The underlying idea was that only medicine could save women from the "horrors" of childbirth. Only white men were allowed access to medicine at this time.

Yet while physicians were busy proselytizing about their medicine, many thousands of women were dying inside of their hospitals. Why? Because physicians weren't washing their hands between patients, and this was causing something called childbed fever to run rampant. Lack of handwashing was shown to be the cause of this fever almost sixty-five years before physicians would agree to handwashing practices.[12]

So maybe now you can start to see how the idea that birth is a "disease-state," or as Dr. Joseph DeLee, a leading obstetric textbook author of the 1920s, put it, a pathologic process from which few escape "damage,"[13] was born. Because there was infection. And people were dying. But what is left out of that story, is the why. (It's worth noting that childbed fever rates were much lower for those giving birth at home.)

Even still, at hospitals and in physicians' care, the standard became to shave the pubic hair, give an enema, sedate, drug, cut the perineal area (see pg 151), deliver with forceps, extract the placenta, medicate again, and repair the cut—in order to maintain as much control over the process as possible to protect against infection.

The mindset that it was safer and more important to control the birth process than care for the wellbeing of our birthing people continued through the 1970s, with extreme medical "solutions" including intense medication, twilight sleep, sedatives, and restraints (such as being kept in cage-like beds and put in strait jackets while in labor—no exaggeration!). Through this time, only about nine percent of medical students were women, which means even fewer were working as OBGYNs, and even fewer of those were women of color.

In following this storyline, it's no wonder so many of us are so petrified of giving birth!

While this was the landscape in America, in Europe midwives were being trained in conjunction with physicians. There was an attempt to introduce this practice in the United States too, but federal funding was denied. Midwives here were still seen as, in the words of one physician, "filthy and ignorant,"[14] even though as far back as the mid-1920s studies show they could have better outcomes than physicians.[15]

Even when midwives did start organizing, the American Academy of Family Physicians (AAFP) opposed nurse-midwifery and issued formal statements through the early 1990s that all nurse-midwives should work non-independently and all payments should go through the physician. Doctors who did participate in home births by offering backups in emergencies were threatened with loss of hospital privileges and even their medical licenses.[16]

Which brings us back to the modern day. Multiple studies show that for low-risk birthers who have access to emergency medical treatments, planned home birth with a trained clinical provider is just as safe as hospital births.[17] Yet the American College of Obstetricians and Gynecologists (ACOG) has published guidelines for how to talk pregnant women out of a home birth.[18] While studies show that states that utilize more midwives have better maternal and infant outcomes,[19] only about eight percent of Americans utilize midwifery care.

While the methodologies may have changed (we are no longer putting pregnant people in strait jackets, though it is worth noting that prisons still use shackles in childbirth), we can still see remnants of our past in how our practices are carried out today.

At present, the US has a cesarean rate of almost double what the World Health Organization recommends[20] and forty-one percent of birthers say their practitioner tried to induce them.[21]

The mindset still exists that controlling birth is the only way to ensure best outcomes—even if the evidence suggests otherwise; even if it means sacrificing birthing people's rights to bodily autonomy and consent; and even if it means jeopardizing their physical and emotional wellbeing throughout the process.

Okay. Whoa! Exhale. Let's pause for a sec. That's a lot of information to take in.

We don't share this to freak you out, or to suggest that birthing in a hospital today is unsafe. An overwhelming majority of Americans birth in hospitals, and we must recognize that this same history is also how we got the very important, lifesaving tools and medicines we benefit from today.

We share this information with you to highlight where the friction in our current system stems from, why so few Americans know what a midwife actually does, and where our cultural fear of childbirth originated.

We share this with you to remind you of your own power. Because if you are reading this book, you likely have the privilege of choice. And while there is so much about this process we can't control, what we can control are the providers we choose to support us through the experience.

Consumer demand is powerful—it is how physicians proliferated in the first place. As a consumer, you get to define the standard of care you are willing or not willing to accept. You don't need to accept a doctor or midwife who makes you feel inadequate, doesn't include you in your care, voices stupid remarks about your family unit, looks at you differently because of your accent or the color of your skin, or doesn't have time for your questions, simply because you trust that person's clinical advice. There are plenty of other amazing clinical providers out there. By accepting that kind of care, you are signaling that that type of care is acceptable. And what we accept is what spreads. So keep reading! We will guide you through weeding out the providers that may create more roadblocks instead of helping you clear your path (see pg 40).

But first, one more thing. We also share this as a way to emphasize the real need to learn how to *tune in*. Because while research is very important, we can't ignore that it is steeped in a history of racism and sexism (plus, it is expensive to fund—so there aren't studies for everything—takes a long time to publish—so the most up-to-date info may not be readily available yet—and is not always representative of all communities and populations). It will also never be able to account for the unique circumstances, the *collections*, of each individual participant—or measure all outcomes.

So while all the research and the resulting institutional policies should absolutely not be ignored, they must be regarded as one piece of the puzzle. And what is the other very essential piece?

You.

Because even with the best provider possible, they will never be able to have full access to your *collection* or to your Gut, Emotions, Body, and Head. And that is very valuable information. That is your superpower.

So now let's meet the most vital concept in this entire book.

INDIVIDUAL DECISION-MAKING

Individual decision-making begins with trusting that you understand what you need. It means taking outside information as a possibility, as information or an option to consider, rather than a must-do. It means *tuning in* and using the information you find inside yourself *together* with the research and advice of your provider and support team.

Whatever person you entrust with your clinical care, their job is to help guide you in your *individual decision-making* process. Your clinician's role should be to assist you in better understanding the research, the measurements, and the numbers, as they apply to your unique Body and circumstances. You and your clinical care provider are a team, and just as you honor and respect their guidance, they need to honor and respect the vital information that you hold. You are both experts at different parts of the perinatal and birthing process.

It's kind of like when Google Maps tells you to go one direction, but you know there is a better way not showing on their database. With that in mind, the following exercise will allow you to check in and see how you feel about your current clinical team. If you don't yet have a care team, consider using these questions as guidelines when selecting your providers.

Ask yourself the following questions about your clinical care providers:

- Do I feel listened to?

- Do I trust their clinical advice?

- Do they include me in conversations around my body? Do they ask *me* questions?

- Do they ask for permission before they touch my body or do any procedure? Do they explain a procedure before they do it?

- Do I feel like they push me into things?

- Do they try and suppress my worries by saying things like "you're fine" or "just don't worry about that" or "we'll talk about that later," instead of trying to understand where my worry is coming from or giving me information that can actually put me at ease?

- Do I trust they will advocate for me?

- Do I feel like they are around to support me postpartum?

In addition, it is vital to ensure that you and your practitioner have the same values—remember that just because you love their personality doesn't mean your values are aligned! To get a better sense of how your values align, go to pg 194, where you will find questions to start the conversation with your birth location and provider.

A very important note: It is rarely ever too late to switch providers. It may be a pain in the butt, but it may also be really, really worth it—listen to yourself on this one!

Before we continue, know that the history we have outlined primarily covers the narrative of colonial white North America, as the source of our current institutions. We would be remiss in not pointing out that birth and reproductive health looked different for enslaved folks and people of color post-slavery, particularly in the American South and other rural areas where midwifery care and the granny midwife retained prominence for a much longer period. (See page 248 for resources on learning more about this very important history.)

GETTING SUPPORT: BUILDING YOUR SQUAD

Now that you have—or are ready to have—your clinical care set up, let's talk through what the rest of your dream team can look like.

Here are some questions you can ask yourself to make sure you'll have the help you need. Note any gaps and areas where you might need extra or a different kind of support.

Pregnancy Support

MY PEOPLE

- Who can help me with my Emotions?
- Who can help me with my Body?
- If I have questions throughout this process, who will I call?

ARE THEY MY DREAM TEAM?

- Do I feel guilty for taking up their time?
- Do they put me at the center of their care?
- Do they make me feel like what I have to say is important?

Birth Support

MY PEOPLE

- In addition to my clinical care team, who else is going to be supporting me during my birth?

ARE THEY MY DREAM TEAM?

- Do I trust them to help me through emotionally?
- Do I trust them to help keep the setting feeling calm?
- Do I trust them to advocate for me if I can't?
- Do I trust them to help me *tune in* when I feel stuck?
- Do I trust them to help me with *individual decision-making* throughout the process?

Postpartum Support

THE EXPERIENCE

- Will I be at home or will I be in the hospital for the first few days? What do I need to support either scenario?
- When and how often will I see my clinical provider?

MY PEOPLE

- Who is going to be my baby's clinical provider?
- Who can I call if I have questions about my baby?
- Who can I call if I have questions about myself?
- Who can I call if I have questions about feeding?
- Who can help me with my Body?
- Who can help me with my Emotions?
- Who can help me with my baby so that I can rest and take care of myself?
- Who can help me with basic household needs (e.g., walk the dog, get groceries, do laundry . . .)?
- Who can help make me meals or organize a meal train for me?

- Who can help me with transit to get to appointments as needed?
- Who can help with my transition back to work?

ARE THEY MY DREAM TEAM?

- Will they be able to support my feeding choices?
- Are they able to support me in *individual decision-making* instead of making me feel like I'm doing things "wrong" even if it is not intentional on their part?
- Am I going to feel like I need to take care of them instead of the other way around?
- Do I feel comfortable doing what I need to do around them?

If you are not sure how to fill any of the gaps that have come up when answering these questions or ensure that you have the appropriate team, see page 202 for our suggestions!

GETTING SUPPORT: WORKING THROUGH THOSE EXTRA BLOCKS FOR LGBTQ+ FOLKS

Those who identify as LGBTQ+ may face some barriers that cis hetero people don't have.

We asked fellow birth practitioners and spouses Morgane Richardson and Alexandra Garcia of Woven Bodies (wovenbodies.com) to share some special considerations to help work through those blocks. These words come from them.

BLOCK: OMG, People Will Not Stop Asking Me Questions about How I Got Pregnant!

Expecting queer parents can look forward to having random straight folks ask them invasive questions about the conception process.

- "How many times did it take to get pregnant?"
- "But . . . how did you *do* it?"
- "Who is the mother/father?"
- "Was it expensive?"
- "Did it hurt?"

Sure, you could open up and tell them all the intimate details—but you don't have to! Remember, most people would never ask these questions of expectant parents who read as straight/cis. So consider arming yourself in advance with some easy answers to nip this in the bud. Come up with your own, or try these:

- "That's a really personal question, so I'm not going to get into that."
- "I'm the parent. There was a donor/surrogate."
- "How did you get pregnant? Like, what position did *you* use?"

Keep in mind, this will likely continue into the postpartum period, even among your own friends and community. You'll start to develop your own flare in how to respond, but don't be afraid to make and accept changes in relationships. This is a delicate time full of beauty and chaos; ain't nobody got time for people who don't treat this period with the utmost respect.

BLOCK: We've Got Hella Extra Financial Stress Because Savings Were Spent on the Conception Process.

Becoming a parent can take up a whole lot of resources when you're queer: money, time, and mental space. While we're over here dropping a couple of G's to introduce the sperm to the egg, sometimes our straight friends don't realize just what an investment it really is.

- Remember that it's normal to have some feelings around this financial reality. It sucks!

- It's okay to take time away from people in your community who trigger negative feelings around this inequity.

- Try to actively schedule into your calendar some free activities you enjoy each week—reading, cooking, taking a hot bath, guilty pleasure TV time—these activities can work to break up cycles of stress. Respect these scheduling commitments just like you would a business meeting or social commitment.

BLOCK: Speaking of Money, Not Only Did I Have to Throw Down Some Cash to Create Our Family; I Have to Pay to Do a Second-Parent Adoption?!

First, let's go into a bit of background on the logistics here: a second-parent adoption is a legal process that allows a parent to adopt their partner's biological or adoptive child, without terminating the first parent's legal status as a parent. While some states recognize LGBTQ+ parents named on the birth certificate, this is currently not the case everywhere in the United States. In fact, some states prohibit second-parent adoption all together!

It's all a bit confusing—and messed up!—and to make matters worse, the laws are constantly changing and family law varies from state to state. So we highly encourage you to look up the second-parent adoption laws in your area and find out what they entail. For example: What rights are assumed at birth? Do you have to do a home visit with a social worker? What are the costs involved?

Depending on where you live, you may or may not have to shell out more cash to do a second-parent adoption, or you might decide to do so even if your state recognizes your family, just to be covered everywhere. But it's not only about the money for a lawyer and social worker—it's also upsetting to go through this process. We encourage you to find a community you can talk to about this to. Your straight friends may not understand, but that doesn't mean you're alone in this.

BLOCK: What If My Family Does Not Acknowledge My Child(ren)?

No matter who you are—straight, gay, gender nonconforming, butch, fem, cis—family dynamics will more likely than not go through a notable change when the baby is born. As a new parent, there's no time to sweat people who don't appreciate how spectacular your new family unit is—it's their loss if they choose not to participate. When thinking about building your Dream Team (see pg 199), you may want to consider seeking out queer and trans–friendly or focused squad members.

BLOCK: I'm Scared I Might End Up with the Homophobic Staff at My Birthing Location . . .

Not all hospitals or birthing places are equipped to support queer families. All sorts of nonsense can come up with uneducated staff, even if it's well intended. If you feel safe doing so, be clear with staff about how you want to be referred to

46

as parents (e.g., mom and mama; john and jane; pops and dad and baba, etc.). Inform the hospital of your rights when it comes to birth certificates and room access, and know that you can report inappropriate staff to the hospital social worker or ombudsman (yep, that's a real job!). We'll go more into your rights as a pregnant person on pg 51.

BLOCK: I'm Not the Gestational Parent. Can I Really Understand the Baby's Needs If I Didn't Birth Them?

Each parent has a unique relationship with the child. The more we can lean into that truth, the more we can support each parent's strengths.

Set the groundwork to feel confident in participating in this relationship. Take a newborn care class. Read some books on infant sleep and development. This can allow you to build your own routine for soothing the baby and playing with them in the first weeks.

Be involved in the prep work. Do the fun stuff like decorating the nursery and choosing clothes, but also get in on the logistics: help organize the clothing drawer, know the pediatrician's name and phone number, know what health insurance the baby is on[22] and whether that needs to change before the first doctor's visit, be fluent in the use of your car seat/stroller. This preparation will allow you to be an active and visible participant in the role of parent as you go out into the world as a family.

This is a new relationship. Like any relationship it takes time to develop. So it's okay not to intuitively know all the answers right from the start. Be patient with the relationship. Give you and your baby time to get to know each other.

That said, this is *your* baby, so go ahead and dive right in with the daily activities. Get involved. Even if you're not nursing, there are tons of ways to create your own special traditions and bonds. Change diapers, do bath time, schedule and attend pediatric appointments. It's in all the mundane little activities that you two get to know each other and learn how to be together.

In cases where the person who carried the pregnancy will also be parenting, try to create a safe space to bring up concerns about equal participation and gateway parenting—where one parent seems to be overseeing the role of the other. Consider some therapy sessions before the baby arrives to talk about how to have these conversations in the postpartum period.

Your extended community of relatives, friends, etc., will be looking to the parents for cues on how to understand the role of the nongestational parent. It's helpful to provide a unified front that clearly says we are both *real* parents.

BLOCK: We're about to Bring This Kid into a Hard World, Especially for Queer/ Transgender/POC Folks.

We could write a whole book on this topic, but in the interest of space we'll leave you with this takeaway: We need more people like us out there asking the big questions, expanding our families, making our voices louder and louder. But while you may have the freedom or desire to speak up for your family—"We're here and we're queer!"—your kids will have to make the conscious decision about whether or not they want or feel safe to come out as a queer family.

It pains us to say this, but you will not be able to protect your child from all of the ugliness and the isms of the world. You can, however, surround them with communities that love and support them. You can teach your kids that they are powerful and supply them with the tools they need to learn when it is safe to speak up and how to do so if they so choose.

BLOCK: Gender Norms Keep Being Peddled by My Surrounding Community. Should I Move?

Sure, it's superimportant to think seriously about what kind of community you might gain by moving. But the reality is that as a broader society we're deeply immersed in ideas and stereotypes of how one should be performing gender—it's everywhere! The cool news is, you're the parent here, so you get to decide how you talk about and perform gender with your family. Trash those cheesy "Dad's greatest moments" photo albums. Read gender-inclusive books, or mix up the pronouns during read-alouds. Let it be known that you are happy to accept all hand-me-downs, regardless of color, cut, or pattern. Live *your* life, not the life someone else wants you to live—by doing so, you'll be setting an example for others to feel safer to follow! So should you move? The decision is ultimately up to you, but if you don't feel comfortable or safe in your home and pushing the boundaries isn't feeling right, then perhaps it's time to find a new community.

PUTTING IT ALL TOGETHER: THIS IS *YOUR* BIRTHDAY PARTY. YOU'RE THE BOSS.

Whoa, that was a journey!

Now that you've gotten in touch with your compass and considered your support system, here is where we encourage you to use your voice and speak up. We don't want you to suffer your way through this very special transition.

As much as we wish people could read our minds and our Emotions, it doesn't always work like that. So please, please ask for what you need as much as you can—particularly leading up to and during the birthing process. If you don't know what, exactly, you need at any point, that's okay. Your support team may be able to help! And sometimes, simply saying you are stuck, unsure, or scared—essentially sharing whatever noise is happening in your Head—may be enough to push through it.

But we know it can be hard to speak up, particularly if you are birthing in a hospital or birth center where you are out of your domain (oh yeah, and you're naked and in labor!). But remember that your provider *works for you*. You are literally paying their paycheck. You are their boss.

With that, we want to remind you of your rights as a pregnant person—because you've got 'em!

#BrilliantTIP

If you are birthing in a hospital, you will be asked to sign a consent form, giving your provider and the hospital staff the right to treat you. This *does not* mean you are giving away your right to informed consent. You still get to consent *every step of the way* and should go through the process described below before you sign any new consent form (for anesthesia, surgery. etc.).

Some of Your Rights*:

YOUR RIGHT TO BODILY AUTONOMY: No one gets to do anything to your body without your permission. Your baby is legally part of your body until they are born.

YOUR RIGHT TO FAIR AND EQUAL TREATMENT: You have the right to be treated as any other patient regardless of your race, age, religion, sexuality, etc.

YOUR RIGHT TO INFORMED CONSENT AND REFUSAL: Before a medical professional can legally touch your body or treat it in any way, they have to participate in a process with you that ensures that they have consent and that that consent was freely given on the basis of information about your clinical condition and the treatments available. It should include three steps:

1 **Inform.** Your provider gives you objective, fact-based information about the condition and the evidence behind the treatment risks and alternatives.

2 **Advise.** Your provider gives you their subjective opinion—what they think is the best course of action.

3 **Support.** Your provider has an ethical obligation and legal duty to support your choice even if it goes against their medical advice (e.g., they cannot withdraw care if you don't follow their advice).

If at any point you feel your rights are being violated, you can ask for a new nurse, a new doctor or midwife, or ask to speak to the hospital administrator or ombudsman.

Check your state's full Patient Bill of Rights.

part
2

THIS IS WHY YOU'RE BOSS: THE CRAZY COOL SHIT YOUR BODY CAN DO

NOW YOU HAVE SOME TOOLS TO START LETTING YOUR BODY, GUT, AND Emotions lead you. You have also thought through your support squad and have the tools to assemble a group that will help you trust that you can *tune in.* With those elements in place, we want to feed your Head new information about your Body so that it can be at ease as it starts to take the back seat during labor.

Your Body was designed to protect you and help you find homeostasis or balance. Every one of your systems was designed for this task; they work on endless cycles, pump blood without vacation time, and take in and filter oxygen while you don't have to move a finger.

All of those processes are so much work! And so, sometimes the Body needs a little—or a lot—of help to get there, and sometimes it just can't make it. But that doesn't mean that your body is broken or that you are not strong enough. It's simply not always possible for the Body to keep up, especially during pregnancy and birth, when it has been working double time for you—and will continue to do so until you stop lactating. By trusting in and supporting your Body, you can actually help it work better and make it easier for it to lead the way.

This section is all about building up that trust between you and your Body. We will show you the brilliant defense mechanisms and communication skills your Body has in place to help you along the way and how you're intrinsically designed to birth your baby and be a parent.

As you'll learn in these pages, it's important to remember there are two bodies at play here: *yours and the baby's.* You're a team! And as difficult as it can be, sometimes, babies know best. They may decide to be born early, show signs that surgery may be safer than a vaginal birth, or position their heads in your pelvis in a way that makes labor and pushing much longer and harder than you anticipated. Or sometimes, your Body will have needs that are different than what you may have expected or hoped for. As we outline how extraordinary this process is and help you build trust, our hope is that you'll know when to speak up if something doesn't feel quite right. And always remember: *while we can influence, we can't control!*

So let's do it! Let's meet all your Body's parts that have helped you so far and those that will continue to help you along the way into the postpartum period and beyond!

We recognize that for some, getting and staying pregnant may have been a very difficult journey. Miscarriages, stillbirths, and the need for assisted reproductive technologies can all make this whole "trusting your body" thing seem impossible. However you got here, we're so glad you made it. The good news is that what follows in this chapter is true no matter your journey to get to this place.

YOUR BODY HAS BEEN PREPPING FOR THIS FROM THE BEGINNING

For many of us, just *thinking* about our periods can be triggering—your favorite white pants ruined, horrible acne, crippling pain, or even a feeling of disconnection from your Body.

But our periods can actually give us lots of information about our overall health—so much so that in 2015, the American College of Obstetricians and Gynecologists called menstruation a "vital sign" alongside blood pressure, pulse rate, temperature, and rate of respiration. Our periods serve as a useful reminder that our Bodies have been practicing for pregnancy for many years.

Our cycles are dependent upon our hormones, and in today's world, it is very easy for our hormones to go haywire. So if you needed a little help to get pregnant, know you're not alone, there is nothing wrong with you, and you are *not* broken. Try instead to think of the assistance as a tool that helped you rebalance. Your Body has been practicing too!

The Breakdown of How Your Body Has Been Practicing

✳ YOUR UTERUS WAS MADE FOR THIS.

Each and every cycle, your uterus works tirelessly to build up its inner layer so that if fertilization occurs it is ready to support implantation. If fertilization doesn't happen, the uterus sheds the lining—that's your period blood—and the process starts all over again. Not only is your uterus smart enough to get rid of what it no longer needs (#lifelesson); it is also crazy resilient. Your uterus grows a whole new lining after shedding the previous one, *just in case* there's better luck next time or the time after that . . . When implantation does occur, your uterus is certainly ready to finally get to build a home for your babe, even if it needs a little outside help to get going (#tinyhouse).

Oh, and those period cramps you may have been experiencing for years? They are actually uterine contractions! They help your uterine lining move from the uterus, through the cervix, and out of the vagina. During labor, uterine contractions are how you will get your baby to move from the uterus, through the cervix, and out of the vagina. NBD. (See pg 75 for more on contractions.) So, while menstrual cramps and active labor contractions may certainly feel different, it can be a nice reminder that this whole uterine contraction thing isn't entirely new for you.

✳ YOUR CERVIX ALREADY KNOWS HOW TO OPEN.

Maybe you've heard that you must "get to 10" in order for your baby to be born. This is referring to your cervix dilating or opening to approximately ten centimeters or four inches (see pg 80) in order for baby's head to fit through. That's a whole lot of opening! But this isn't a new trick for your cervix. Your cervix has actually been opening and changing with every cycle since your very first period. During ovulation—when the egg is released—the cervix softens, lifts higher in the body to make it easier for fertilization to occur, and opens slightly for sperm to enter. Then it closes back up. When you bleed, the cervix opens again and lowers in the body to help the uterine lining flow more easily out of the vagina. And then it closes again.

YOUR VAGINA HAS A BLACK BELT.

Ever wonder what's up with that white stuff in your underwear? That's your cervical fluid, and it's proof that your vagina is stellar at self-defense. It is also proof that your vagina is very capable of protecting your baby. The cervical fluid does two very important things: One, prior to pregnancy, your cervical fluid changes consistency throughout your cycle (maybe you've noticed sometimes it's more watery and other times more globby or stretchy) to either help (around ovulation) or prevent (all other times) sperm from being able to reach the egg. Sperm won't survive without your fluid helping it along. Two, the fluid carries out dead cells and bacteria to guard against infection.

You may notice you've had increased fluid during your pregnancy—this is your body working overtime to cleanse and protect itself. The mechanism by which your body produces this fluid is similar to how your mucus plug is created (see pg 60)

THIS ISN'T THE FIRST TIME YOUR VAGINA HAS GROWN.

During orgasms, the vagina becomes engorged—aka the vaginal walls flood with blood and cause the vagina to grow in size.[23] So, your vagina has been growing and shrinking since the beginning of your sexual life (or at least every time you O).

YOUR MILK GLANDS HAVE BEEN ACTIVATED BEFORE . . .

Your milk glands are activated during *every* cycle since you first got your period! Your breasts/chest changes throughout the cycle, practicing for lactation. When you bleed, your milk glands (see pg 91) enlarge in case fertilization occurs when you next ovulate. (This is why you may feel like your chest is lumpier during this time.) As you inch toward ovulation, your milk ducts (see pg 91) also grow. If no fertilization occurs, the stimulation of your milk glands will just start all over again.

THIS IS HOW YOU GROW A BABY: NEW WAYS TO THINK ABOUT YOUR CHANGING BODY

Now that you have a sense of how your body has been prepping for pregnancy, let's talk through the new superpowers that you develop once you are actually pregnant.

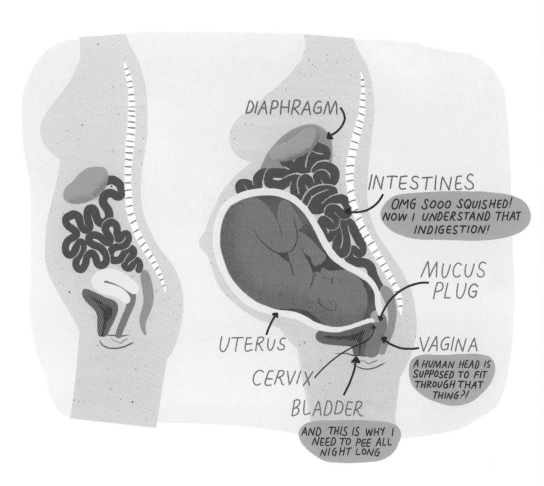

58

Check out that difference! No wonder the side effects of growing a human being can be so rough sometimes. But as you down those antacids, know this: The same changes that may be torturing you during pregnancy are also allowing you to sustain a home to grow and nourish your baby—and not just any home, but one that is flexible and amendable—shifting and changing as your baby develops to best fit its needs. Now this doesn't mean you can't be psyched to give the baby its "eviction notice" when the time comes, but in the meantime, here are some incredible new ways in which your Body is supporting you.

Some of Your Superpowers

- **Your blood volume increases almost 50 percent so that enough nutrients and oxygen can get to your babe.**[24]
  This helps account for that swelling (not fun!), but it may also allow for some amazing orgasms thanks to increased blood flow to the genital area (more fun!).

- **Your diaphragm and ribs change position so you can breathe in more oxygen for baby.**
  While you may feel short of breath sometimes, you are actually able to take in more oxygen while pregnant! Your diaphragm literally lifts, and your rib position changes, allowing for an increased capacity to breathe in more air.[25]

- **You make a mucus plug.**
  Delicious sounding, we know. But your cervix creates this barrier in the beginning of your pregnancy—at around four weeks—to block bacteria and other invaders from getting inside.

- **Your uterine vascular system gets an entire remodel.**
  The volume of the uterus will expand about 500 times during pregnancy[26] (eee!). As a result, your uterine veins and arteries will *physically enlarge* to help with the extra flow. If only all home remodeling were this easy!

- **Your vagina stretches.**
  To answer the question—yes, a human head *can* fit through that thing! And it's all thanks to your vaginal rugae—transverse ridges that allow the vagina to be elastic and resilient. Gotta love those rugae! If you are worried about the vagina, well, shrinking back, see pg 163.

- **You get more white blood cells to help fight infection and platelets to help with clotting.**
  These numbers increase more dramatically as you approach labor and they stick around through the postpartum period to keep you safe and help you heal![27]

- **Your breasts/chest change so baby can more easily find them.**
  You may notice that your nipples stick out more, become darker, and the small bumps around them, more pronounced. All of these changes are thought to help your baby find your breast/chest once born. The darkening makes it easier for your baby to see your nipples, and those bumps, called Montgomery glands, secrete a multipurpose oil that keeps things moist—thank you very much—and releases a scent that draws baby to the nipple.

A Note on Your Changing Body: Weight Gain

While this is all truly wondrous, we recognize that all this change can also be overwhelming, both physically and emotionally. We also know that care providers can add to this stress by putting a lot of emphasis on your weight. There are many factors that contribute to a healthy pregnancy: blood sugar levels, blood pressure, sleep, stress, and nutrition, just to name a few. To get a real understanding of your health, you must look at the whole picture, not just what the scale says. If you feel your provider is putting a lot of emphasis on your weight, ask about your other health indicators to get a sense of where their concern is coming from. If the added pressure feels unwarranted and/or unwelcome, remember you can always switch providers!

For your own sanity, when you're feeling like a whale, remember this: You are *actually* carrying a bunch of extra weight around. And it's not just the weight of your baby. Here's a breakdown, in pounds, of all your added cargo:

BLOOD = **3** pounds

BREASTS/CHEST = **2** pounds

WOMB = **2** pounds

BABY = **7.5** pounds (toward the end of the pregnancy)

PLACENTA = **1.5** pounds

AMNIOTIC FLUID = **2** pounds

FAT, PROTEIN, AND OTHER NUTRIENTS = **7** pounds

RETAINED WATER = **4** pounds

From March of Dimes, based on averages.

MEET YOUR HORMONES

So much change! How does it all happen? In large part, it's thanks to major shifts in your hormones.

Our relationship to hormones is funny. Roars and cries and chin pimples are typically what come to mind when we think of "being hormonal." We often forget that those amazing feelings of warmth, joy, and pure pleasure are also caused by our hormones. We also forget that they are central to almost every bodily function we have! Hormones are our chemical messengers, delivering the information that tells all of our parts what to do.

Hormones have helped you immensely in growing your babe thus far, and so it should come as no surprise that they are also central to labor, postpartum recovery, and your ability to lactate.

So let us introduce you to some of the major players in the perinatal period.

Estrogen + Progesterone

These two often work as a team!

WHY THEY'RE AWESOME

- They help you maintain a safe uterus to house your growing babe. That thick uterine lining is thanks to them.[28]

- They activate painkilling pathways in your brain and spinal cord to give you an epidural au naturel while in labor.[29] (More on this ahead.)

- They help your breasts/chest prepare for lactation.

- Progesterone prevents the uterus from contracting during pregnancy.[30]

- Progesterone helps loosen up the joints to ease the passage of baby through the pelvis.

- Estrogen builds a whole wiring system of oxytocin receptors inside the uterus, which in turn allow the uterus to contract during labor and postpartum.[31]

- Estrogen also stimulates the release of prostaglandins[32] (see below) to start softening the cervix so that it can dilate—aka open—for baby to be born.

- Estrogen promotes blood flow and lubrication to the vagina and vulva and keeps the vaginal tissues elastic so they can stretch as baby comes through.

#BrilliantBIT

During pregnancy progesterone levels are ten to eighteen times higher than they were pre-pregnancy. And estrogen levels go up by more than a thousand times, with a peak right before labor starts.[33] This is why you feel all the feels!

Prostaglandins

Technically, these are not exactly hormones, but we included them here because they are known to have hormone-like effects and they work hard to prep your body for labor.

WHY THEY ARE AWESOME

- Leading up to labor, prostaglandins help your cervix soften and get more elastic so that it can open more easily.

- They help stimulate and relax the uterus to prep it for labor.

- They give you the pre-labor poops by stimulating the GI tract to help you clear some space[34] #babycomingthrough.

- Once labor gets going, prostaglandins increase the sensitivity of the uterus to oxytocin to help with contractions.[35]

Oxytocin

The hormone of love, baby!

WHY IT'S AWESOME

- Oxytocin triggers all kinds of useful contractions. We know this doesn't sound so awesome, but read on!

  - Oxytocin is what causes your uterus to contract in labor (see pg 68). You may hate it for this, but remember, *contractions are what allow your baby to be born!*

  - Oxytocin will help your uterus contract after the birth to protect you against postpartum hemorrhage and to help get your uterus back to its pre-pregnancy shape and size. We know—you thought you were done! But these *do not* feel like labor contractions, don't worry! (See pg 74 for more info.)

  - Your milk ducts (see pg 91) need to contract as well for your milk letdown to happen. As baby sucks on your nipples, your body produces oxytocin, which causes those contractions![37]

- It gives you and baby the warm fuzzies!

  - You know that sensation of deliciousness when you hug someone you love, eat chocolate, or snuggle with a puppy? That's your oxytocin at work. When your baby is born, you'll get the biggest burst of oxytocin in your lifetime![38] (Partners can experience this burst too.) This oxytocin kick will help you bond with your baby. And your babe gets a burst too,[39] making them feel safer and calmer when you snuggle them.

- Oxytocin can also reduce anxiety and stress when you breast/chest-feed,[40] which can make those feeding sessions more pleasurable for you and the baby.

#BrilliantBIT

Oxytocin is also the hormone responsible for orgasms! Because of this, there are some people who actually experience orgasms during the child-birth process.

Beta-endorphins (BEs)

Our natural painkillers.

WHY THEY'RE AWESOME

- They reduce stress and produce feelings of euphoria and pleasure[41] that help you cope with labor's sensations.[42] Some people even report feeling like they entered an altered state of consciousness while in labor—aka they feel *high*. This is thanks to those BEs. #signmeup.

- After baby is born, the BEs stimulate your "reward center," which can help you feel pleasure when you come in contact with your baby.[43]

- They facilitate the release of prolactin,[44] the hormone that produces milk.

> ### #Brilliant BIT
> There are also BEs in your colostrum (early milk) to help your newborn cope with the stress of the postpartum transition.[45]

> ### #Brilliant TIP
> We know you may not want to, but exercise throughout your pregnancy if it's medically possible. Studies have shown that regular exercise in pregnancy may enhance BEs during labor![46]

Catecholamines

Catecholamines are also known as adrenaline and noradrenaline (or epinephrine and norepinephrine). These hormones protect you if you're in danger and help you cross the finish line.

WHY THEY'RE AWESOME

- If you aren't safe during labor, these hormones can stimulate the fight-or-flight response (see below) to slow down or halt your labor so that you don't give birth in a dangerous environment.[47]

- Catecholamines peak right before you start pushing to give you the extra oomph you'll need to push your baby out.[48] They then drop once baby is born[49] so that you can chill and rest with the little one.

> ### #Brilliant BIT
> If you feel afraid during labor, sometimes your catecholamines can kick into gear, causing your labor to pause even if you're not actually in danger. If you are birthing in a hospital, this can happen in transit or when you first get to triage because of the change of environment, especially if you aren't in active labor yet. See pg 118 for more on stalled labor.

66

Relaxin

Relaxin relaxes your tissues, joints, and ligaments so you can create lots of space in your body to make room to birth your babe.

WHY IT'S AWESOME

- During pregnancy, it relaxes the uterus so it can stretch as baby grows and expands.

- It relaxes your blood vessels to increase oxygen to the placenta—so baby can "breathe"—and the kidneys—so you can get rid of all that extra waste.[50]

- In preparation for birth, it softens the pelvic joints and ligaments making the pelvis more flexible.[51] (See pg 82.)

- During labor, it softens and relaxes the cervix by relaxin' it (hehe) and allowing it to stretch and open.

Prolactin

The *pro-lactation* hormone.

WHY IT'S AWESOME

- This hormone triggers milk production! Prolactin starts kicking in around the 20th week of your pregnancy—you are actually making milk while pregnant!

- Prolactin ups your appetite during pregnancy and while lactating to make sure you get the calories[52] you'll need.

- It reduces stress by stimulating oxytocin and endorphins while you nurse,[53] which allows us to feel good when we feed our babies.

- It gives you a feeling of submission and surrender[54]—that parental instinct to put your baby first. #bossbaby

67

Putting It All Together

Now that you know how each hormone plays its part, here's a very simplified version of how the whole orchestra works together during labor.

While no one knows exactly how labor begins, what we do know is that at the start of labor estrogen levels go up, signaling an increase in oxytocin receptor sites on the uterus. This uptick causes the prostaglandins to increase so the cervix can soften and the uterus can get ready for that oxytocin to come. Oxytocin is pumped through the blood causing the uterus to contract as it comes into contact with the oxytocin receptors. Those contractions cause BEs to be released so that you can cope with the sensations. And the cycle continues (see pg 76 for the contraction feedback loop) until baby is ready to be born, at which point there is a surge in catecholamines so that baby can be "ejected." When baby is born, oxytocin peaks and catecholamines decline so you can rest and enjoy snuggles. When the placenta is born progesterone drops, which increases prolactin levels to help you feed your babe.

Curtain closes.

Please note: What is described above is what happens in physiological labor— meaning when the Body is left to do its thing without interventions. Interventions— like inductions, an epidural, or Pitocin, for example (see pg 136)—are introduced in order to mimic this physiological process. Sometimes they are just the ticket the body needs to revamp or jump-start the labor conversation. But other times, because they are synthetic and because there isn't a medicine that can actually regulate the number of hormonal receptors your body has, they can stifle communication or not be effective.

WELCOME TO YOUR BABY'S HOME—THAT YOU FREAKIN' MADE FROM SCRATCH!

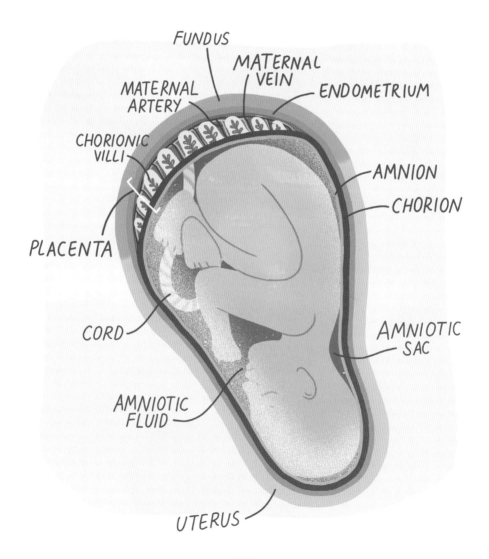

Placenta

Okay, not only did you grow a baby, but you also grew an entire extra organ—one that will weigh about 1.5 pounds, be approximately the size of a dinner plate, and even produce its own hormones.

The placenta is a big deal. It is the site of all communication and exchange between you and your baby. What are you exchanging? Blood—and through it nutrients, antibodies, oxygen (your baby isn't breathing with its lungs yet—all the oxygen comes from *your* bloodstream see pg 16), and waste.

#BrilliantBIT

Although the placenta prevents "mixing blood," research is now showing that your baby's cells can still cross the placenta barrier and enter your body. #babygonerogue. Baby's cells can become your liver cells, muscle cells—they can even cross the blood-brain barrier and turn into your neurons![55] So bits of your baby stay in you forever and parts of you are still in your mom!

#BrilliantBIT

While the placenta here is pictured above the baby, sometimes the placenta grows in front of baby, and sometimes behind or even below. When the placenta is in front, it's called an anterior placenta and generally not concerning or problematic. In those cases it's normal to feel less movement and kicks as it's almost like you have a cushion softening the blows between you and the baby. If the placenta is below the baby, it is possible for it to cover part or all of the cervix. Sometimes the placenta can move out of the way, but if it doesn't, this becomes an indication for a cesarean, as the gateway for baby to get out is being blocked.

Amniotic Sac + Fluid

Together, these provide your baby with the ultimate security during development. The sac is formed by two membranes: the amnion, which more directly contains the fluid, and the chorion, which connects to the placenta. The two membranes slide over one another to reduce friction and therefore breakage as the baby twists and turns in the womb (#greatdesign). The chorion also contains chorionic villi—microscopic, fingerlike projections that help absorb extra nutrients for the babe as well as ensure that your blood stays separate during pregnancy.

The amniotic fluid—which by week 20 is mostly made of your baby's pee, along with antibodies, hormones, and nutrients (#orginalvitaminwater)—serves as a shock absorber to protect baby from the outside world. It also helps protect them in their inside world by maintaining a regular spa-like temperature and keeping the umbilical cord from becoming compressed. The amniotic fluid allows babies to prepare for the outside world by working out their digestive system as they swallow it and by strengthening their muscles and bones as they swim around.

Cord

The umbilical cord is the tube that attaches you, via the placenta, to your baby, through a small hole in their soon-to-be belly button (#TheMatrix). The cord is the tunnel through which everything the placenta lets into the womb travels to the baby. And baby's waste must travel back through the cord to be disposed of by the pregnant person. It's a two-way highway in there! The cord can grow to be almost two feet long and has a jelly-like covering, called Wharton's jelly, which helps prevent it from kinking.

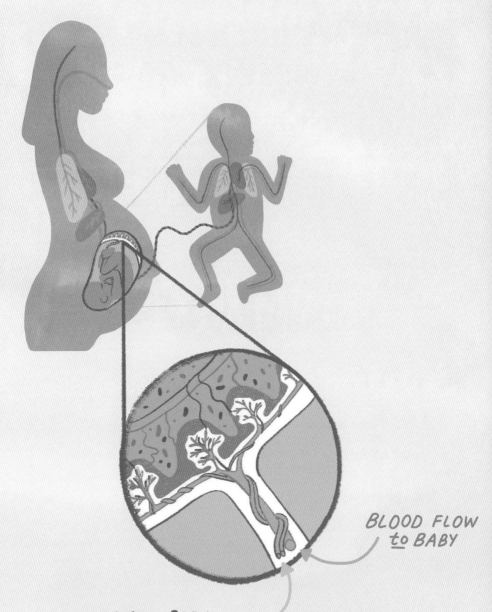

BLOOD FLOW to BABY

WASTE from BABY BACK TO PREGNANT PERSON TO GET RID OF

#BrilliantTIP

Once baby is born, you can ask your provider to delay clamping and cutting the cord until it is done pulsing. This generally takes a few minutes, but it is less about exactly how many minutes you wait and more about ensuring baby is getting all the blood that's still in the placenta before the connection is lost. This increases your baby's blood volume and iron storage levels, makes their transition to breathing with their lungs easier, and can help prevent future issues like anemia and also assist with brain development.[56] [57]

#BrilliantBIT

Contrary to popular belief, it is actually very common—and generally not dangerous, thanks to that Wharton's jelly—for the cord to be wrapped around the baby's neck! In fact, it occurs in about one-third of pregnancies.[58] Sometimes, it is even wrapped around multiple times!

THE UTERUS: OH HOW IT GROWS (AND SHRINKS!)

The uterus is an amazing organ. Its capacity to grow, stretch, and accommodate weight is truly outstanding.

As you may have learned from a pregnancy tracking app, your uterus will have gone from the size of a small pear to the size of a watermelon by term. Take that in for a second. Your uterus will have gone from weighing about 0.06–0.22 pounds and living deep inside of your pelvis to weighing about 2 pounds[59]—not including the baby's weight, amniotic fluid weight, or anything else!—and extending from the pubic area to the bottom of your rib cage!

But wait. We're not finished! After doing all that work in pregnancy, the uterus still has a big job to do even after baby is born. The uterus will need to continue contracting post-baby to encourage your placenta to peel off the uterine wall and come out of your vagina—usually about 5–45 minutes after baby. Once the uterus is done with all that birthing, it has the brand-new job of contracting back to its pre-pregnancy size and location in a process called involution.

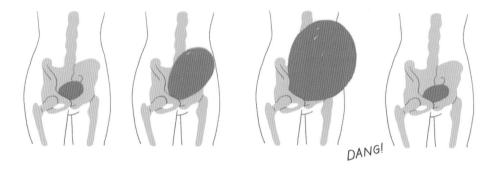

DANG!

HOW IS THE UTERUS SO FLEXIBLE?

Thanks to the hormone relaxin (see pg 67), increased blood flow, and the specific smooth muscle and tissue makeup of the uterus, it is able to stretch and thin, kind of like a balloon.

HOW DOES IT SHRINK BACK?

All that oxytocin and the postpartum contractions shrink the uterus back to size. Remember all that uterine vascular remodeling? Well, no baby means no need for extra blood flow. So the postpartum contractions help constrict the uterine blood vessels to prevent excessive bleeding. Without that added blood flow and with all the contractions, the uterus will shrink back down to pre-pregnancy size and snuggle back into your pelvis. During this process, your body will need to rid itself of the by-products of your healing womb. You will see blood and tissue leaving your vagina for up to around six weeks postpartum, regardless of whether you had a vaginal or surgical birth. This bleeding is called lochia, and it is a sign that your body is healing.

#BrilliantBIT
Breast/chest-feeding will help your uterus contract as it activates oxytocin production!

DO POSTPARTUM CONTRACTIONS HURT?

For some they can be intense for the first few days. This is particularly true if it is not your first birth, as the uterus needs to work a bit harder after being stretched out again. Laying flat on your belly with a heating pad, keeping your bladder empty, and hot showers can be helpful. Your provider can also offer you pain medication.

HOW DO I KNOW IF MY UTERUS IS NOT SHRINKING PROPERLY?

If you are giving birth in a hospital, the average provider will not see you again for six weeks after you are discharged. A lot can happen before then! This puts the onus on each of us to ensure we are checking in and watching out for signs of irregularities. And for those who see their providers sooner, it is still important you check in with yourself. Watch for excessive bleeding and trust your Gut. If at any time you feel off or are not sure of your status, it's always better to call your care provider.

THE UTERUS: DEMYSTIFYING THOSE CONTRACTIONS

Now that you have a sense of your uterus's many talents, let's talk about one more . . . *contractions!*

Don't run and hide! What we've found is that the more you understand what is actually happening to your body during a contraction, the easier it will be to cope with them and accept them as they come and go.

The Dance

Contractions work on a positive feedback loop, meaning contractions themselves are what signal for more contractions to come. This loop is often described as occurring in a wave-like pattern: You feel the sensation of a contraction begin to build until it peaks, and then the sensation begins to come back down. You get a nice little break (thank goodness!) before the sensation starts to build up again.

Here's how the choreography of this feedback loop works to give you that wave-like effect:

(Please note, while this is referring to a baby in a head down position, it works similarly for a breech baby—just different parts in different places)

A contraction is the dance of oxytocin molecules traveling through your bloodstream, landing on oxytocin receptors on your uterus (which have increased dramatically for labor thanks to the extra estrogen and the prostaglandins), and then vacating those receptors, thanks to an enzyme called oxytocinase (made by your placenta!) which quickly metabolizes those oxytocin molecules so that they don't overstay their welcome.[60]

When the contraction happens, the fundus, or the top of the uterus, presses on your baby's butt which in turn, allows for baby's head to press on your cervix. It is this pressure that not only helps the cervix to open (thanks, baby!) but also signals your cervical receptors to tell your brain to send more oxytocin to your uterus for the loop to continue.

There is a period of time when the old oxytocin molecules have vacated the receptors and the new oxytocin molecules haven't yet replaced them. It is during this period that you get that much needed break between contractions. Phew!

When baby is born, this loop is broken, as pressure is no longer detected by the cervical receptors (since baby's head is no longer there).

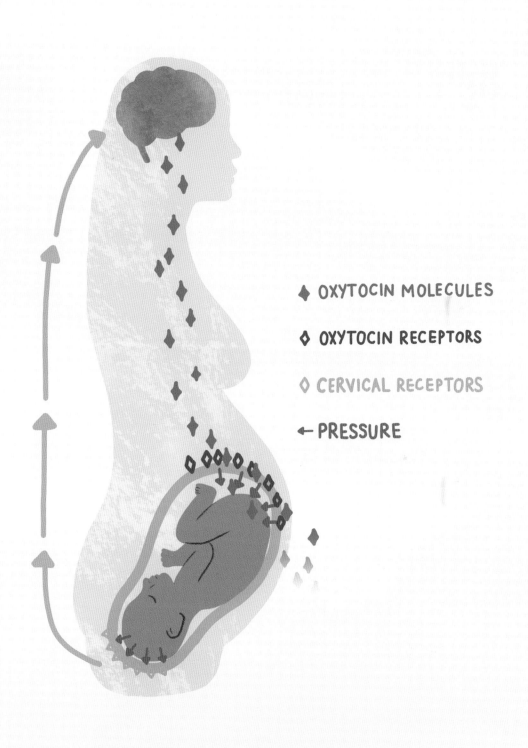

◆ OXYTOCIN MOLECULES

◇ OXYTOCIN RECEPTORS

◇ CERVICAL RECEPTORS

← PRESSURE

Your Uterus Has Got Moves

The uterus is a unique, complex, and intricate collection of different muscle layers that all work together to help your cervix open and expel your babe. So how does it respond when the play button is pressed (aka those oxytocin molecules land in the receptors)?

There is a common misconception that the cervix dilates *out* or is pulled open from side to side. But the truth is that during a contraction, it is actually being lifted *up* and *outta the way* by the different muscles of the uterus.

NO CONTRACTION

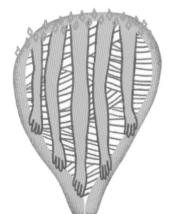

DURING A CONTRACTION

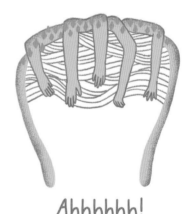

Ahhhhhh!

And all of this heavy lifting isn't in vain. As these muscles move up and out of the way, they don't vacate the dance floor. Instead, they help to build that fundus so it has enough oomph to help get that baby outta there!

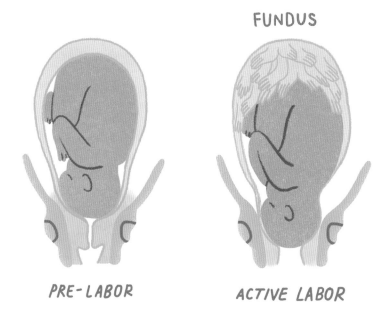

FUNDUS

PRE-LABOR   ACTIVE LABOR

With all this said, it is very helpful to remember that contractions are *productive*. They are happening *with* you and *for* you, not *to* you. When you feel those strong sensations, remind yourself of what you are feeling—you are literally feeling your uterine muscle layers hard at work lifting your cervix up and out of the way so that you can meet your baby.

THE ALMIGHTY CERVIX

So far all of our talk about the cervix has revolved around opening or dilating . . . and don't get us wrong, we think the fact that the cervix can expand to approximately ten centimeters is pretty freaking *wild*. But the cervix deserves *even more* credit. Look at all the other work it has to do too.

IT SHIFTS FORWARD!

The cervix will move from a posterior position, to a more anterior position—allowing your baby better aim down the chute, ya know?

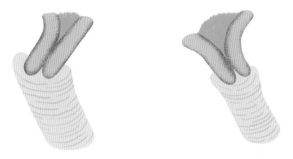

IT GETS SOFTER!

Touch the tip of your nose. Now touch your lip. That is approximately the change your cervix will make throughout labor, in part thanks to those prostaglandins. (See pg 63.)

IT GETS THINNER!

This is also known as *effacement* and is measured in percentages during cervical exams (pg 118)—with 0 percent being still very thick and 100 percent as thin as it can be!

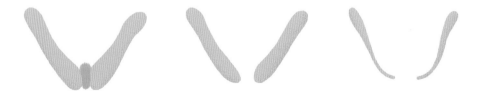

IT GETS SHORTER!

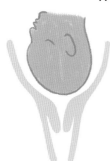 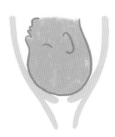

IT OPENS!

Once all of that starts happening, *then* it becomes a lot easier for the cervix to open.

The cervix's journey during the lead-up to birth is a lot like sucking on a Life Savers candy—the longer you suck, the thinner it gets and the wider the hole becomes. While dilation is measured from 0–10 centimeters (0 being totally closed, and 10 being fully open or dilated), the truth is that there is no measuring device used during this process. Your provider is basing your dilation number off of how much cervix they can feel in relation to your baby's head. So if you get exams from two different people, you may get different results solely because their perspectives are different.

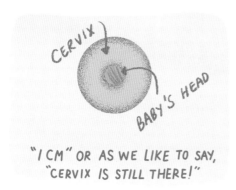 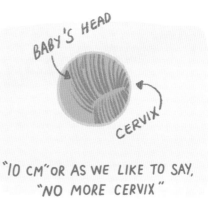

"1 CM" OR AS WE LIKE TO SAY, "CERVIX IS STILL THERE!"

"10 CM" OR AS WE LIKE TO SAY, "NO MORE CERVIX"

See how much work your cervix is doing to help you prepare for that baby to come through?! This is why labor can be so goddamn long!

81

THE PELVIS PART 1:
A PELVIS LIKE ELVIS

Okay. The part you've been waiting for: how is that baby getting out of your body?!

As your body changes during pregnancy, you may notice that your pelvis is changing too. Perhaps your hips feel larger, or maybe one side feels tighter or you're a little wobbly or off-balance when you walk around. These are all signs of the hormone relaxin at work, loosening up those pelvic ligaments to eventually help that tight squeeze out be, well, a little less tight.

#BrilliantBIT
This tight squeeze is actually really good for the babe. When their head is squeezed, they experience a surge in catecholamines, which gets their metabolism going, protects them from low blood sugar, and helps them learn to breathe and regulate heat. And when their chest is squeezed, it works to clear their lungs of amniotic fluid so that they can breathe easier.[61] Cool!

But still, how on earth
does a baby make it through?

Your pelvis helps you out! Look what your pelvis does as baby comes through . . .

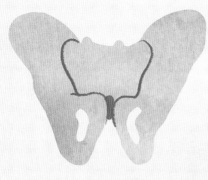

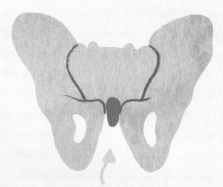

APPLY PRESSURE
TO THESE BADBOYS

IT GETS WIDER!

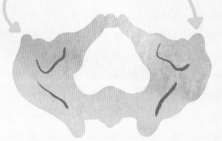

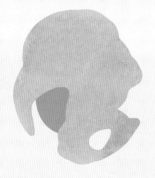

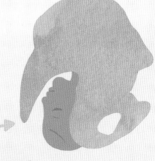

AND VOILÀ! THAT OUTLET
IS MORE SPACIOUS!

THIS SCOOTCHES
OUT OF THE WAY!

Throughout your labor, your practitioner may want to get a sense of where your baby is in relation to your pelvis. This is called your baby's *station,* and it is a measurement of where the presenting part (either the head in most births or feet or butt in a breech birth) is in relation to the ischial spines of your pelvis. The station is typically measured in numbers from -5 to +5.

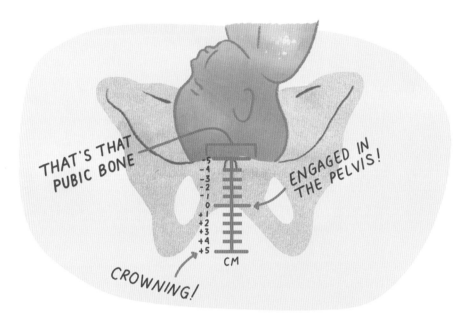

The main takeaway here is that when you are in the negative numbers, baby is not yet locked and loaded in the pelvis. For most full-term babies, 0 station means that baby is engaged. Once we get to the positive numbers, baby is on the descent out! When baby is at +5, their head is visible to the outside world (aka crowning).

It is possible for you to first begin your labor at a positive station. But this doesn't mean your baby is coming any moment! See that big ole pubic bone in the way? That's why pushing can take a few hours, especially if you've never done this before—because baby's head still needs to make its way down and under that bone. See pg 209 for more on pushing phases.

84

THE PELVIS PART 2:
I HAVE A WHAT?! DISCOVER YOUR PELVIC FLOOR.

Check that out! You have an entire hammock of muscles in your pelvis holding everything in place!

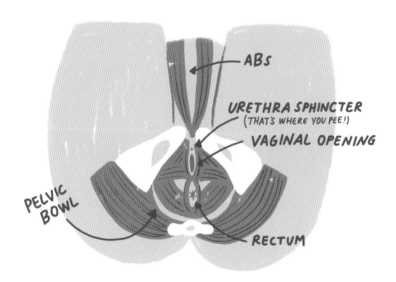

Finding Your Pelvic Floor

Cough and focus on your nether regions. Can you feel your pelvic floor moving up and down? High five!

SO WHAT DOES THE PELVIC FLOOR DO?

You can thank your pelvic floor for four main things:

1. **Supporting your organs.** It helps hold your uterus, bladder, vagina, rectum, and abdominal muscles in place.

2. **Continence.** It helps you, ya know, not pee or poop your pants.

3. **Orgasm.** #enoughsaid.

4. **Stabilization.** Because your pelvic floor is connected to your core, it helps your abs and back have movement control.

HOW IT WORKS

Your pelvic floor is made of a network of muscles, nerves, ligaments, and fasciae. It contracts or relaxes throughout the day, depending upon the activity at hand.

Peeing, pooping, or having penetrative sex? That's your pelvic floor relaxing. Orgasms? That's your pelvic floor contracting. Not peeing your pants? Those muscles are contracting again.

For optimal functioning, the pelvic floor needs to have a full range of motion, meaning it needs to be good at *both* contracting and relaxing. The good news? Your pelvic floor has been practicing contracting and relaxing since your very first breath! Your pelvic floor is connected to your upper abdominal muscles and your diaphragm. This means it moves up and down every time you breathe! Try some deep abdominal breathing. Inhale (it relaxes); exhale (it contracts). Can you feel your pelvic floor moving?

What's Up with Kegels?

Glad you asked! Kegels are an exercise in which you voluntarily contract or tighten your pelvic floor muscles by sucking them upward, like through a straw.

Now, before you go nuts counting how many Kegels you can do on your way to work, let us remind you of the importance of that full range of motion. Kegels are a great way to practice contracting and strengthening the muscles, but not such a great way to practice the release. And for baby to make it through, those muscles need to release! We will leave the contracting to the uterus.

Here's how you can practice releasing your pelvic floor. Take a deep inhale, filling your belly with air. As you feel your belly fill, see if you can also feel that pelvic floor getting wider, expanding—you can even try pushing it out a little in a "reverse Kegel."

The tone of everyone's pelvic floor is different, and it's possible for it to be too tight or too loose in different parts of the hammock. So, if you don't know what's going on with your pelvic floor, continuously Kegeling may not be the best thing for your body. When one part is tighter than the other, baby may need to tilt their head a certain way to compensate, affecting how effectively your baby is able to put pressure on your cervix and fit through your pelvis.

To this end, we highly recommend you see a pelvic floor specialist during your pregnancy, if you can, so that they can offer exercise suggestions based on your unique pelvic floor tone. Webster technique–based chiropractors can help address imbalances (see pg 200).

#BrilliantTIP

Instead of Kegeling, practice abdominal breathing! Because this allows for relaxation *and* contraction, it is a great way to connect with your pelvic floor without creating further imbalances. Unless you know for sure that your pelvic floor needs strengthening, Kegels may not be the best exercise for you in pregnancy.

GOT MILK

Oh hello there, brand-new—and much larger—chest!

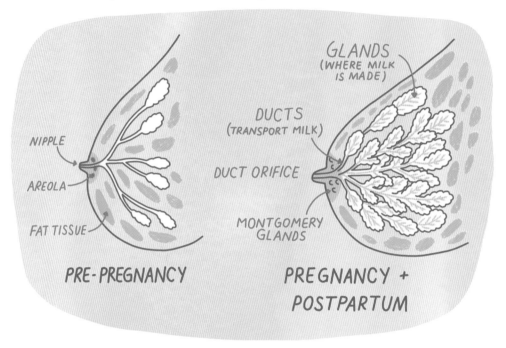

GLANDS
(WHERE MILK
IS MADE)

DUCTS
(TRANSPORT MILK)

NIPPLE

DUCT ORIFICE

AREOLA

FAT TISSUE

MONTGOMERY
GLANDS

PRE-PREGNANCY

PREGNANCY +
POSTPARTUM

#BrilliantBIT
Milk production has nothing to do with the size of your breasts/chest. Big, small, lopsided—they all contain a similar amount of milk-producing tissue.

Okay, get ready. Whether you choose to breast/chest-feed or not, the mechanisms in place to make it happen are pretty freakin' neat.

Remember how tender your breasts/chest felt in the first trimester? Well, that was your ducts and glands at work prepping for lactation. . . . You already have milk! Thanks to the prolactin, when you are around 20 weeks' pregnant, you start producing colostrum, aka your first milk, aka "liquid gold." (Some people may leak during their pregnancy, others may not. If you don't, this doesn't mean that you don't have colostrum.)

Colostrum is all your baby needs for nourishment for the first few days of life before your mature milk comes in, generally around day 3–5 postpartum. Why is it called liquid gold?

- It is thick and goldish and somewhat sticky.
- It is perfectly engineered to be low in fat and high in carbs and proteins so newborns can digest it quickly.
- It has a laxative effect that helps baby poop.
- It helps organize your baby's metabolism and microbiome for later digesting of your mature milk.[62]

Once your mature milk comes in, it is all your baby needs to eat until you start introducing solids—and this includes water! How is this possible you ask? Check out all the things that are inside your mature milk[63] (#smartmilk):

- Water (Breast/chest milk is 88 percent water, which is why you don't need to give baby any extra.)
- Protein
- Lactose
- Essential fatty acids
- Long-chain polyunsaturated fatty acids
- Breast/chest-specific macrophages (a type of white blood cell for immunity)
- Antibodies
- Hormones and growth factors
- Stem cells
- Oligosaccharides (sugar)
- As many as 800 types of bacteria (the original probiotic)
- Antibacterial and antiviral enzymes
- Vitamins and minerals

And get this—the specific composition of your breast/chest milk will change to fit your baby's needs! It's different in the morning than at night, at the start of a feeding than at the end of the same feeding, if baby is sick (it can actually provide antibodies![64]), and as baby grows. It changes depending on your diet and lifestyle.[65] It changes depending on the season[66]. . . we could go on and on.

> ## #BrilliantBIT
> As you produce milk, you're literally melting your own body fat, starting with your butt![67] You'll be burning, on average, an extra 580 calories to produce the amount of milk your baby needs every day,[68] so it's important to continue eating well in the postpartum period.

How does your body know what kind of milk to make? No one is entirely sure. But one theory is that there's a vacuum effect when baby sucks on the nipple, delivering fluids from their mouth—a mix of milk, saliva, maybe even snot (yum!)—back into the milk ducts of the breast/chest.[69] This is thought to give information to your body on what the milk's composition should be for your babe's unique needs at the time.

> ## #BrilliantBIT
> For an extra layer of protection, when your breast/chest milk mixes with baby's saliva, a chemical reaction occurs that produces hydrogen peroxide to prevent the growth of harmful bacteria like salmonella and staphylococcus.[70] And get this, it only happens with *your* baby's saliva—it doesn't happen with adult saliva. Presto!

So How Does Lactation Work?

When your placenta is born, a message is sent to rev up the body's prolactin production. But once this "systems go" signal is sent, it then becomes *your* job to let your body know that it needs to keep the milk factory in business.

Breast/chest-feeding works on a positive feedback loop, meaning, the more you stimulate your nipples by feeding your babe or pumping, the more milk your body knows it needs to make. Stop stimulating your nipples and the body stops making milk. There are two parts to how this loop works: the milk letdown and milk production.

MILK LETDOWN

- Baby sucks on your nipples and stimulates the nerve endings that tell your brain to release oxytocin.

- Oxytocin flows through your bloodstream and into the breasts/chest.

- Tiny muscle cells surrounding your milk glands are squeezed. Remember oxytocin causes muscle to contract!

- Milk is squeezed from the glands into the milk ducts and travels to your nips. Hello letdown!

- Baby sucks the milk out of your nipple.

- This then triggers the stimulation of nerve endings again and thus the loop begins anew!

#BrilliantBIT

When you're not feeding, your duct orifices have valves that close to help prevent milk leakage. But note, these aren't foolproof: you might still leak when your breasts/chest are full.

MILK PRODUCTION[71]

- As baby sucks on your nipple, the stimulation tells your brain to also release prolactin.

- Prolactin travels through the bloodstream and into the breast/chest.

- Prolactin attaches to the prolactin receptors on the walls of the milk glands. When they attach, it triggers milk production.

- When these glands are full of milk, the glandular walls expand, changing the shape of the prolactin receptors so that new prolactin molecules can no longer fit, thus *slowing* milk production.

- As baby drinks and empties the breast/chest, those pro-lactin receptors return to their original shape and prolactin molecules can once again attach themselves, thus triggering milk production again.

Essentially, when your chest is full, milk production slows down. When your boobs are emptier, milk production is faster. This is why constant feeding in the beginning is so important—so your body can get on board that milk train.

Important note: Each side of your chest has its own loop. This means you need to give both sides the same amount of attention; otherwise one side can underproduce while the other overproduces or vice versa.

DON'T FORGET YOUR BABY: IT TAKES TWO

As you can see, there are *so* many ways your body has been programmed to help you through this process. But this doesn't mean the pressure is on to perform! You are not in this alone; your baby is helping you along the way. And not only will babies help you birth them, but they'll help you keep them alive as they transition into this world! They're a lot more resilient than they look.

Here is how baby has developed to help you out.

How Baby Helps While in Utero

- Remember how the Wharton's jelly (see pg 71) helps prevent kinkage in the umbilical cord? Well, baby's movements in your uterus are also helping to keep the cord free-flowin' and preventing the cord vessels from becoming compressed.

- Though baby isn't breathing with lungs in utero, at around 10 weeks babies start prepping their lungs to breathe actual air once born, by moving amniotic fluid in and out.

- Though the exact mechanism of how labor starts is still unknown, it is thought that there is some kind of communication between you and baby that gets it going—but this is still just a theory.

- Remember those catecholamines baby produces? See pg 82. Well, they not only set up metabolism, breathing, and heat regulation, but also help baby learn a birth parent's smell and protect them if the cord gets compressed during contractions.

- Ever wonder what that cheesy-looking white stuff on your brand-new baby's skin is? It's called vernix. This protective layer of grease not only helps insulate baby and protect their skin in the aquatic environment of your uterus, but it also acts as a lubricant as baby descends through the birth canal. Whee!

How Baby Helps You Out, So They Can Get Out!

Despite the pelvis not being quite a straight shot out, babies are usually really good at finding their way. They innately know how to move, rotate, and shift to get to the widest spaces to pass through. In fact, all babies will know how to make roughly the same movements—how insane is that?

These movements are called the seven cardinal movements and typically look something like the illustration on the next page.

Now you know how baby so wisely maneuvers, but you may still be wondering how it is that a human skeleton can make it through another human skeleton without breaking. Turns out, baby's bones are very flexible! Feel the tip of your nose. Go on, feel it! That's what *all* of your baby's bones are like at first because they are mostly made of cartilage. Plus, they are not all fused together yet—most infants have more than 300 bones while adults only have 206! This cartilage will harden into what you typically think of as bones over time.

Baby's skull bones are no exception. Because they are not yet fused together, the skull bones are able to slide over one another, contracting and avoiding damage as they are compressed in the birth canal. This is why babies can have a cone-shaped head when they're born! Don't worry, if that does happen, your baby's head will return to its regular shape soon.

Thanks, baby!

#BrilliantBIT

Here's another incredible way your baby may help you out: Research[72] is showing that fetal cells can be found in birth parents' scar tissues, specifically scars left by C-sections. These cells make collagen. So it's thought that your baby may be helping you recover from your surgery!

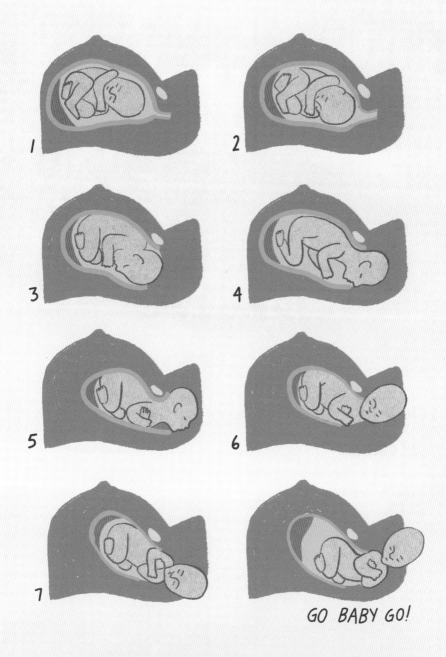

GO BABY GO!

part

3

THE PRENATAL
WHAT-IFS

Hopefully by this point in the book you've accomplished the following:

- You feel confident about your support system.
- You feel clearer on your unique needs and desires for this transition into parenthood and what may be standing in your way.
- You have some tools to cut out the noise and start *tuning in.*
- You have a new understanding of your superpowers and rights as a birthing person.
- You have some newfound trust in your Body's capabilities.

With all this said, we know you probably still have a lot of *"But what ifs . . ."* floating around in your mind. We've got you. This next section is all about addressing the common fears and anxieties around labor and the postpartum period.

It's okay to worry about these things. In fact, they are in this book because *so many people* have these same worries. Just because you think about them, doesn't mean that they will happen to you! Sometimes the best way to protect yourself against those fears taking over is to go there and dive into the information.

Our hope is that this section will give you the info your Head needs for a new perspective on some of your anxieties, as well as the tools to navigate even the worst-case scenarios.

WHAT IF . . .
I DON'T GET THE BIRTH I WANT?

Unlike many other books out there, we are not prepping you to get the birth *you want.* It's actually quite likely that your birth will be very different from what you are expecting. The sensations you will end up feeling will not be what you imagined, you'll love something you thought you'd hate, and you'll hate something you thought you'd love.

None of these things will mean you've "failed" your birth. The most powerful thing you can do in labor is to be able to listen and trust yourself and your needs without judgment—moment to moment (or contraction to contraction), each step of the way . . . *especially* when those needs mean letting go of your "plan." It is this adaptability, this letting go, this knowing and asking for your truest needs, that is the real beauty of birth. That's you owning that compass like a boss.

So instead of helping you get the birth you want, we hope to give you the tools so that you can feel safe within the unknown, move moment to moment, and feel supported around *the birth you end up getting.*

The Real Formula for "the Birth You Want"

1   Make sure you are choosing the clinical team that can actually support you in your preferences and needs and that supports your *individual decision-making* (see pg 39.)

2   Build your *Dream Team* (see pg 199) and use them! Remember, you are not in this alone.

3   Invest time and energy building up a conversation with your Body, Gut, and Emotions. Help your Head feel safer by addressing its concerns (see pg 12).

4   Try to let expectations around your birth experience go. (We know this one is hard!)

5   While you're in your labor, *go inward* throughout (see pg 100).

6   Try not to put too much pressure on yourself to follow a specific path. It doesn't matter what *kind* of birth you have. It only matters that you felt supported and that you were an active participant throughout. Sometimes being kind and forgiving with ourselves is harder and braver than

accomplishing a specific goal. So focus instead on how to best nurture yourself along the way, and ask for help when you aren't sure. What you are doing is a big freakin' deal. And just because so many people do it, doesn't mean it's easy. You are a total badass for going through this. Remind yourself of this over and over again.

#LaborTOOL
GO INWARD

At any point throughout your labor when you feel overwhelmed, stuck, unsure of what you need, or just want a moment to pause, *tune in and go inward*. This is the most important tool to help you moment to moment.

- **Check in with your Head.** What is it saying to you? Can you change the language? Do you have a specific fear or thought your support team may be able to help you with? Speak up! Do you have a question you'd like to ask? Ask!

- **Check in with your Body.** It's a good practice to continue asking yourself, *What do I feel right now?* While you may not be the coziest you've ever been, it'll help you see what sensations you are *actually feeling* (like lower back pain) in relation to what you are *thinking* (like you're afraid of the back pain to come). If at any point there is a felt sensation that is alarming you, tell your support team.

- **Check in with your Emotions.** Is your Head making you feel scared or anxious? Communicate your Emotion. Do you need to release with a cry, laugh, scream, or funny sound? (See pg 213 for Release + Reset tools.)

- **Check in with your Gut.** Do you have a feeling about something? Share with your support team. Is your Gut telling you to move your Body in a certain way? Go with it. Remember—you are not in this alone and you are connected to the millions of birthers that came before you.

WHAT IF . . .
I STAY PREGNANT FOREVER?

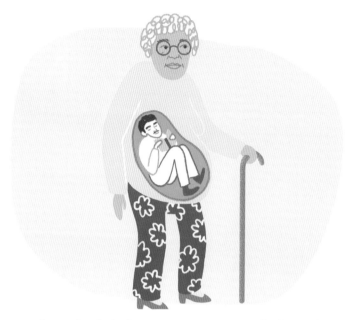

We know you know that baby has to come out eventually. But in those final weeks, it can feel like maybe you'll actually be the first person to have a baby inside of them forever.

We feel you.

Here are some tips to help you stay in the flow.

THINK ABOUT A "DUE MONTH" INSTEAD OF A "DUE DATE."

Your EDD (estimated due date) marks what is supposed to be your 40th week of pregnancy. But, the average first-time parent actually goes into labor *after* 40 weeks.[73] So to help you stay out of the waiting mindset, think about a "due month" instead of a "due date," starting from your 37th week and extending through your 42nd week—you are considered "at term" throughout this window. And plan for the longer run so that your Head doesn't start screaming once you hit your EDD.

KEEP YOUR EDD A SECRET.

As your due date approaches, lots of well-intentioned folks will likely be checking in to ask how you're doing (read: to see if you're *still* pregnant). For some, all this attention is exciting. For others, it can make that giant clock in your head ticktock even louder. So, if you would rather avoid people blowing up your phone, we recommend you skip the details when talking about your due date. You can share what your "due month" is, or be vague when people ask you when you're due: "I'm due late spring!" or "I'm due around Thanksgiving." You get the picture.

HAVE FUN.

That's right. Though this may seem impossible at first read, these are your final days with your family as it currently stands. You're already giving so much of yourself, and you're about to start giving so much more. So take advantage of your last few weeks—or days! Go on dates. Be with friends. Eat delicious foods. Watch movies all day. Do that creative project you've always wanted to. Go to the museum if you are feeling up for it. Walk in the park. Get a massage. Cook. You do you. This is your time. You deserve it! And it'll make time pass quicker.

HELPING YOUR BABY COME SOONER.

Here's the hard but simple truth: no matter what the internet may lead you to believe, you actually don't get to control when the baby comes—unless you schedule a C-section. Practicing letting go of the control here is an important part of the process—as there's a whole lot more you won't be able to control coming your way (hello, parenthood!). The good news? Letting go of control can actually feel so much better. It is easy to get caught up in all the "doing" to get the baby to come that you end up spending your last days even more stressed out and exhausted. If having intercourse would feel nice, do it! If you love acupuncture, go! Is spicy Indian food your fave? Order it on Seamless. But we encourage you to spend these final weeks on *you* instead of focusing on all the things that are *on you* to do. The baby will come, we promise! If you are facing an induction if your baby doesn't come by a certain time, keep reading.

WHAT IF . . .
I'M TOLD I NEED TO BE INDUCED?

In one survey, four out of ten birthers (41 percent) in the United States said that their care provider tried to induce their labor.[74] So, it's no wonder if this is a concern of yours! The following are some tools to help you navigate the induction conversation if it comes up once you are near term. Partners and support people, take notes! It's your job to help advocate on behalf of the pregnant individual.

The most common reasons for inductions in pregnant people that are considered low-risk and have no health complications include:

- You are past your due date and still pregnant.
- The baby's size is a concern.
- The amniotic fluid levels are either too high or too low.[75]

Ironically, despite the list above being the most common reasons for induction, they are not always evidence-based—meaning, either the research available doesn't show that outcomes are *necessarily* better and/or there are other factors that haven't been taken into account in the studies, like margins for calculation errors and weighing the *risks* of having an induction against the *benefits* of waiting for labor to occur on its own.

#BrilliantBIT

Inductions may also be recommended to ensure you end up with a certain care provider at your birth. Remember, your care provider will not be in the room for most of the time. You do not need to plan *your* birth around your practitioner!

When You're Told You Need an Induction . . . But You Don't Feel Ready or Aren't Sure It's Medically Indicated

When an induction is recommended, it is totally normal to feel a little scared. Take a couple deep long breaths. Inductions can take a few days before the baby is actually born. So if it were a true medical emergency, you'd likely be going to the operating room. Inductions are often more a preventative measure—it would be safer for baby to be born sooner—than an immediate emergency!

ASK YOUR PROVIDER

- Why are you recommending an induction?

- Do I have any other risk factors?

- Is baby's health okay *today*?

- Is there anything about my health that is concerning you *today*?

- How ready is my body for an induction? Based on my cervical exam, what is the likelihood that the induction will be successful? (This is measured in something called a Bishop Score.)

- What happens if I don't get induced?

- Can I have a few more days?

- Would it be safe to continue my pregnancy and wait for me to go into labor on my own if I come in for regular checkups?

#Brilliant TIP

Remember, you can never be forced into an induction—you have the right to refuse, no matter what. If you're not comfortable with the decision or want a little more time, it's okay to say you're not ready. Even if your care provider is making you put a date on the books or they claim they "don't have a slot" for you later on, it's still your right.

What to Do If You're Told . . .

YOU ARE TOO FAR PAST YOUR EDD.

These days it is really common for hospital-based providers to start talking about inductions close to 40 weeks, if not sooner. Evidence does show the best outcomes occur when baby is born by 42 weeks, but it also shows that there is no clear right or wrong path if you are induced at 41 or 42 weeks.[76] So hello, *individual decision-making*! Talk to your provider about your preferences, goals, values, and how ready (or not ready) your body is to give birth.

#BrilliantBIT

Make sure your EDD (estimated due date) is correct! If you know when you conceived or when you typically ovulate, and think your EDD may be off, this is important to talk through with your practitioner as it could have implications on when an induction is recommended and how far past your due date you actually are. If you have a longer cycle (which can make your EDD off by a full week!) or didn't have a sonogram in your first trimester (which is the most accurate way to calculate it) you might want to talk to your practitioner about your EDD.

YOUR BABY IS TOO BIG OR TOO SMALL.

To start with, you can always ask to be remeasured. The ultrasounds that typically determine the baby's size are notoriously off. In fact, ultrasounds can fall anywhere from 15 percent above or below the baby's actual weight."[77] In one study, one out of three people were told that their babies were too big, but the average birth weight of those babies turned out to only be 7 pounds, 13 ounces which is very close to the average birth weight overall of babies born in the U. S.[78]

A "big baby" isn't actually an evidence-based reason for an induction.[79] Remember all the cool moves your pelvis can do? Those are meant to accommodate your baby's size, even if it's a bit on the larger end of the spectrum. So, in the event of a "big baby," you can simply refuse induction if there are no other evidence-based concerns on the part of your provider/care team.

If baby is measuring small, it is important to have a discussion with your provider about how baby has grown *over time,* not just about the current measurement. This way you can get an understanding of whether it looks like baby's growth is actually being restricted—which would be an evidence-based concern—or if baby is simply just measuring on the smaller side while everything else looks good.

YOU HAVE LOW/HIGH AMNIOTIC FLUID LEVELS.

If an induction is being suggested due to low or high amniotic fluid levels, ask to be retested. While fluid levels can be an evidence-based reason to be induced, these tests are also not foolproof. A second test is a good way to prevent making a decision on false reads.

Amniotic fluid levels are directly related to your hydration, so if you're told that your fluids are too low, be sure to drink a ton of water between tests. If your providers don't want you to go home and come back before being retested, ask if they can give you IV fluids beforehand. If, after being retested, the levels are still concerning, then you can more confidently make your decision with the added information that it wasn't a false read or just dehydration.

When an Induction Is the Right Next Step for You

Here are some tips to keep the birthday party fresh!

ASK YOUR PROVIDER HOW IT WILL GO DOWN.

There are different methods of induction depending upon where you are giving birth and the readiness of your body to start. Ask your provider to walk you through step-by-step how they plan on inducing you so that you can feel a bit more prepared. Also ask when and what you will be able to eat throughout the process, so you can plan accordingly.

GO HOME FIRST.

If it is not a scheduled induction, go home before heading to the hospital. This will give you a chance to digest the change of plans, ground yourself, and prepare a little more physically and emotionally. Take a warm shower, listen to your favorite tunes, etc. Again, inductions are more preventative measures than emergencies, so let yourself have some time.

EAT.

In many cases, you may not be able to eat for much of your time in the hospital before baby is born. So be sure to have a nice meal before you head on over. We also recommend bringing snacks with you to the hospital.

PLAN FOR THE LONG RUN.

Inductions can take hours, or they can take days. It's important to wrap your head around the fact that you may be in the hospital for a while. Remember—there's so much your body needs to do to be ready to give birth, so give yourself the time you need.

BRING THE FUN WITH YOU.

Since inductions can be quite long, bring some fun with you so that you don't get trapped in that "waiting around" feeling. Bring an iPad or laptop so you can have movies, games, music, apps, and podcasts all at your fingertips . . . Mix it up! It can also be nice to bring some vibes to the room to make it feel homey—think flameless candles, photos, trinkets.

GET OUT OF THE BED WHEN YOU CAN.

As important as rest is throughout the process, your baby still needs to find their way down into your pelvis, so it's very important to keep yourself moving to help encourage baby to do so. See pg 214 and 218. Don't just lay in bed if you don't have to!

> **#BrilliantTIP**
> Gestational diabetes is another very common reason for inductions. If your GD is under control without insulin, your baby is measuring healthy, and you have no other risk factors, then there is mixed research and recommendations to support inductions.[80] So if avoiding an induction is really important to you, it's important to have a conversation with your care provider—ideally in advance so that you can express your wishes early on.

WHAT IF . . .
MY WATER BREAKS ON MY BOSS'S SHOE?

The thought of fluid pouring out of your vagina in a public place is no fun, particularly at work and in front of people you will certainly have to see again.

Let's talk it all through.

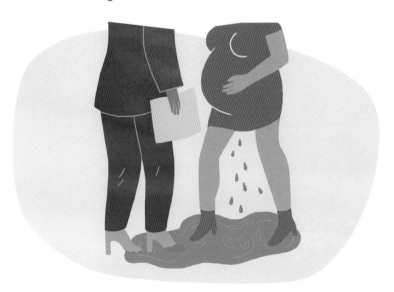

IT'S ACTUALLY NOT COMMON.

The good news is that contrary to what the movies may lead you to believe, your water breaking as the first sign of labor—meaning before you start having contractions—only happens in about 8–10 percent of pregnancies.[81] Most people's water doesn't break until they are having consistent, strong contractions, and for some, it never breaks at all. This means that most of the time, you'll already know you are in labor and will have plenty of time to get home before you wet yourself.

IF IT DOES HAPPEN, YOU WON'T ALWAYS SOAK YOURSELF.

This is another big misconception we can thank Hollywood for. Not everyone's water breaks in a big ole gush. For some, it can feel like a trickle—leaving you confused as to whether your water actually broke, you're experiencing a high volume of vaginal discharge, or you have just peed yourself. This means that the chances of anyone else knowing that your water has broken is even less than 8–10 percent. If you aren't sure your water has broken, check in with your provider or doula.

IS THE THOUGHT STILL TRIPPING YOU UP? TAKE SIMPLE STEPS.

If the thought of your water breaking in public is very distressing to you, you can consider wearing a light pad toward the end of your pregnancy, just in case, or bringing some with you when you're out and about. We've even had clients bring a spare pair of leggings and underwear in their bag. In the very, very, *very* slight chance that your water does gush onto your boss's shoe, consider them blessed. After all, that very fluid is how they got here!

IT DOESN'T MEAN YOUR BABY IS COMING!

Many people falsely believe that as soon as the water breaks, they need to rush to the hospital because the baby is about to be born. If this is your first time giving birth and your water breaks but you are not experiencing strong, consistent contractions, it could still be a full day or two before your baby is born. This means that your water breaking is not necessarily an indication to head to your birthing place straightaway. (More on this below.)

If you *have* given birth vaginally before, things *can* move quickly from here, so be sure to check in with your provider right away.

#BrilliantBIT

Once your water breaks, you will continue to leak amniotic fluid until baby is born (so you may want to put on a pad and put a towel down beneath you so you don't ruin a couch). But don't worry, baby is still safe and protected. You'll continue to make more fluid and you'll never release every last drop. However, it is important to stay superhydrated! Remember, the fluid is mostly baby's pee at this point, so the more you drink, the more baby pees, and the more the fluid is replenished.

#BrilliantTIP

No matter when your water breaks, be sure to check the color. Your amniotic fluid should be clear and odorless—although it's okay if there is a tinge of blood in it. If you notice green, yellow, or brown in your fluid, it is likely an indication that baby has pooped inside you—baby's poop is called meconium, or mec for short. If you think you may have some mec in your fluid, don't freak out. Often this is NBD—even babies in utero gotta go. But, because meconium can also be a sign of distress, it is important to let your provider know as soon as you see it.

Prepping Just in Case Your Water Breaks Before You Experience Contractions

It is important to have a conversation with your care provider before you're at term (37 weeks) to get on the same page in case you do find yourself in this situation. It's *way* easier to have the convo before you're *in it*.

The plan for how to proceed will likely be different depending upon your GBS or strep B status. If you do test positive, know that it is not an STI and you are not diseased. GBS is an innocuous bacteria that about one in four pregnant people in the United States carry.[82] Although it's totally harmless for adults, there is a slight chance it could be passed on to baby, and then an even slighter chance baby might become infected by it. And if this happens, it can make the baby very sick. When your water breaks, the risk of exposure is heightened, though this does not mean that your baby will become infected. It just means you'll need to head to your birthing place or let your care provider know sooner rather than later. Your practitioner may want to take preventative measures by giving you antibiotics.

If you are GBS negative, most hospital-based providers will still want your baby to be born within twenty-four hours of your water breaking to guard against infection. But research shows that so long as your fluids are clear and you have no other risk factors, evidence supports both inducing labor in this situation or allowing the pregnant person to wait for contractions to begin at home for up to 2–3 days.[83] Because these are both evidence-based options, this is where your *individual decision-making* comes into play. This is particularly important for those who are hoping for an unmedicated birth or fewer interventions, because if you go to the hospital too soon, your chances of interventions increase. If you are birthing at home or at a birthing center, the protocol is to give your body the time it needs, unless there are medical indications otherwise.

#BrilliantTIP

Regardless of your GBS status, if your water breaks, you can reduce your risk of infection by not putting anything in your vagina—no douching, fingers, penis, toys, etc.—and staying very hydrated,.

WHAT IF . . .
I GIVE BIRTH IN THE CAR?

This is such a common fear, probably because those taxi-born babies always make it to the news. But it's actually extremely rare . . . like 0.07-something percent![84]

But since this fear comes up so often, here is some more information to put you at ease.

KNOW WHEN TO GO.

Unless you have another plan with your provider for a specific reason, the best time to go to your birth place is when you are in active labor. Clinically, active labor is when you are at least six centimeters, but because you can't do cervical exams at home, there are other signs you can watch for that can be helpful indicators (see pg 203 for more on stages of labor). If you are working with a doula, they should be able to help you assess when to go.

- **A 3-1-1 contraction pattern.** Contractions are coming every three minutes starting from the beginning of the last contraction, each contraction is lasting for at least one whole minute, and this pattern has been happening for *at least* one whole hour.

- **Bloody show.** As your cervix opens, you might start seeing some bright red blood, not too dissimilar from period blood. This is not the same as the mucus plug, which, though it can be blood-tinged, it is thick and globby and looks more like snot than your period.

- **Pressure in your butt.** As baby comes down through the pelvis, you'll start feeling like you're going to poop your pants—this can be a great sign of your body getting ready to push.

Each one of these on their own isn't necessarily an indication of active labor. If *two* of these are true for you, it might be a good idea to head on over to your birth place, if you aren't there already.

PUSHING TAKES A WHILE!

Even if it feels like your baby is coming, it is helpful to know that it can still take hours before the baby is actually born. So even if you start having the *urge to push* in the car, you still likely have time to get there.

#BrilliantBIT

The pushing phase—well, most of labor actually—typically goes a lot quicker if you've had a vaginal birth before. Remember, the likelihood of you having that baby in the car is still around 0.07-something percent—we did the math!—but you will likely want to head to your birth place sooner if this is not your first rodeo. This is a conversation you should have with your provider *before* you get close to the end of your pregnancy.

#BrilliantTIP

If you *really* feel like baby is coming, put your fingers into your vagina and see if you can feel baby's head. If you can't, that's reassuring! If you can, stay where you are or pull off the road, call 911, and do your thing. If baby comes before anyone else gets there, just guide baby toward your chest—don't pull. And be sure to keep baby warm once born—skin to skin if possible and put a jacket or something over them. Don't cut or pull the cord and don't get up until the medics come.

PLAN AHEAD.

It's important to consider how fast you can get to your birth place or the nearest hospital, because even if you're planning a home birth, there's always a chance you might have to transfer. So plan your drive. How are you getting there? How long is it going to take? What is the quickest way to get there? Who's driving?

Do you want your partner/support person to drive or do you want them helping you in the back seat? If they are driving, will they be able to find parking easily, or does that mean you'll have to enter your birthing place alone? Having a solid transit plan will ease some of the anxiety around the commute.

How to Stay in the Flow While in Transit

No lies here—a car ride while in active labor can suck. But here are some ideas that might make the transition to your birth place a little smoother:

- Ask the driver to take it easy. There's no need to run red lights or drive like a maniac.

- Sitting may not work for you. Getting on all fours or leaning over the back seat may be more manageable.

- Keep it cozy. Bring some pillows to lean on.

- Keep it clean. If your water has broken, you may want to lay a towel down beneath you.

- Tune out. Close your eyes, listen to some music with headphones, wear an eye mask.

- Pee before you leave. You won't want to be trapped in the car with a full bladder.

- Doggy style it. Sometimes putting your head out the window and feeling the air on your face can feel nice.

- Bring a full water bottle to stay hydrated along the way.

WHAT IF . . .
MY BABY IS TOO BIG?

Toward the end of pregnancy it can feel like there's a cow growing inside you.

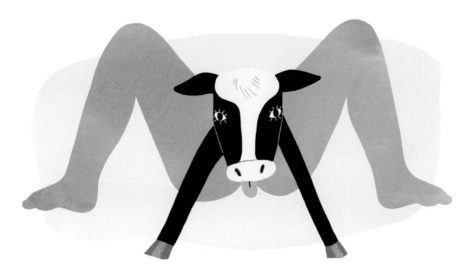

And it may be hard to fathom how the hell this thing is going to come out. If your baby is measuring on the bigger side, we know this feeling can be intensified, particularly if you are getting constant reminders from your practitioner or hearing all those "OMG your belly is huge" comments from well-intentioned folks.

So, let's talk through this whole "big baby" thing.

WHAT'S TECHNICALLY A BIG BABY ANYWAY?

According to the American College of Obstetricians and Gynecologists, a baby is considered big—medically called macrosomia—if the estimated fetal weight is greater than 4,500 grams (9 pounds, 15 ounces).[85]

REMEMBER, WEIGHTS ARE ESTIMATES!

According to the Listening to Mothers Survey,[86] one out of three babies are estimated to be "too big" at the end of pregnancy, when in reality only about one in ten babies is born "large."[87] The only way to really know how big or small your baby is, is to weigh them *after* they are born.

IF MY BABY MEASURES BIG, WILL I NEED A C-SECTION?

Although a lot of providers tend to recommend planned cesareans for suspected big babies, there is actually no significant evidence that confirms that the benefits of surgery outweigh the benefits of a vaginal birth, when you weigh in the risks of cesarean births.[88] When there are no other risk factors or health history considerations, the recommendation to OBGYNs from ACOG is to offer (not recommend) cesareans to people without gestational diabetes whose babies are estimated to weigh over 11 pounds and to people with gestational diabetes whose babies are estimated to weigh over 9.9 pounds.[89] But remember, *individual decision-making!* You can always opt out of surgery, and conversely, if, for whatever reason, you don't feel like a vaginal birth is the safest choice for you, opting for a cesarean birth is also your right and a valid choice.

IF MY BABY MEASURES BIG, WILL I NEED TO BE INDUCED?

Similarly, there is no strong research that supports inductions for suspected big babies. In fact, this can actually make it more difficult to birth your baby, as inductions can limit your ability to move around and create more space in the pelvis for baby to come through. Inductions also increase the likelihood that you will use an epidural if you weren't planning on it already, which not only limits your ability to move around during labor but also limits the positions you can push in.

IS IT POSSIBLE FOR MY BABY TO ACTUALLY JUST NOT FIT?

Most of the concern over bigger babies actually stems from practitioners' fear of shoulder dystocia, or when baby's shoulders get stuck while coming through the canal. While this can certainly be scary, it is actually impossible to predict the majority of shoulder dystocias. Only about 7–15 percent of big babies have trouble birthing their shoulders,[90] and at least half of the cases reported of shoulder dystocia happen in smaller babies.[91] There are certain factors that put you at higher risk outside of baby's estimated weight, so we encourage you to have a discussion with your practitioner if this is a concern, so you can make an informed choice for your unique situation.

True cephalopelvic disproportion or CPD, is when the baby's head or body is *actually* too big to fit through the birthing person's pelvis. This is extremely rare and usually limited to those who have experienced extreme malnutrition, were diagnosed with rickets, are pregnant at a very young age, or have had a pelvic injury.[92] Many times, if baby is having trouble making it through the canal, it is because of the *position* or *angle* of baby's head, not size.

Things to Remember about Your Baby Being "Too Big" to Fit

- The pelvis shape isn't fixed! By applying pressure in certain places, stretching, and doing certain movements, you can actually make the pelvis roomier (see pg 218).

- Baby's head isn't fixed either. Not only is baby's head malleable (see pg 94), it can also change angles and positions throughout labor and pushing.

- Pushing positions matter! Pushing in different positions—like squatting, trying both sides, and on all fours—can help create more space in your pelvis for baby to come through.

WHAT IF . . .
MY LABOR STALLS?

It's no fun feeling like you're stuck. And if you are birthing at a hospital, the language you may hear doesn't help matters: *"You're failing to progress." "You're only three centimeters." "You have a lazy uterus."* Though we can't control what people say, we *can* reframe what "progress" really means. The truth is that it's literally impossible for you *to not be* moving forward while you are in labor! As time passes, you are moving closer to birthing your baby no matter how long it takes, even if there are some breaks in the process.

Here are some tools to help you remember that you're always moving forward.

THE CERVICAL EXAM

Throughout your labor, you will likely have cervical exams. This is your provider's way of getting a sense of where you are in your labor. From the birthing person's perspective, these exams can feel like . . . exams! *Did I progress enough? Is four centimeters a good enough result?* Oh, the pressure!

During a cervical exam, your provider is looking for a few different things:

1. **Effacement** (see pg 80)

2. **Dilation** (see pg 81)

3. **Station** (see pg 82)

4. **Cervical position** (see pg 80)

5. **Consistency** (soft/medium/hard)

Yet often, practitioners will only share the dilation information with you. This is a huge disservice to you as a patient, because those other measurements matter in understanding how your body has changed over time. There is nothing worse than working your butt off contracting for three hours and then hearing you haven't changed in dilation. Asking about your *station, effacement, cervical position,* and *cervical consistency* will give you more information about what's really happening. Your dilation may not have changed, but the other indicators may have!

#BrilliantTIP

Remember, there are no real measuring devices for these exams. So whenever possible, see if you can get the same person to perform them each time. This way you can have a more nuanced discussion of how your body has changed, since the practitioner will have their experience with you to pull from, not just numbers on a piece of paper. This will also help prevent against "backward reads" due to practitioner discrepancies. No one wants to hear they are at three centimeters after being told hours before they were at four!

In addition to asking about all the indicators above, we also recommend you ask about:

Baby's Position: Your provider might be able to determine which way your baby is facing in your pelvis, or if baby's head is tilted. Sometimes the position of baby's head can prolong labor (see pg 122), so this information can clue you in to whether you need to try and create more space in your pelvis for baby to turn (see pg 218).

IT'S NOT ALL ABOUT THE NUMBERS.

It's easy to get caught up in the numbers as the gold standard to tell us how we are advancing. But progress in labor can't always be measured in this way. The information you receive from a cervical exam will only tell you where you are, not where you are going. We've seen people go from three to ten centimeters in three hours, and we've seen people take three hours to get from eight to nine centimeters. There's no way of knowing what will come. So, try not to let exams make you feel discouraged.

#BrilliantTIP

If the numbers from your exam will psyche you out, you can always ask your provider not to share them.

#LaborTOOL

We encourage you to stop using your Head to think about progress in terms of time and numbers, and instead focus on your Body. Here's how:

The Self-Exam

With every physical exam, ask yourself the following:

- Do my contractions feel different from when I last did a self-exam? Are they stronger? Are they lasting longer? Are they coming closer together? Are they slowing down?
- Do I feel pressure in a new part of my body?
- Has my Emotional state shifted?
- Have I seen new fluids or blood?
- Was I able to give my body some good rest?

It's almost impossible you'll feel exactly the same as you did the last time you checked in with yourself. This is a nice reminder that labor is never static!

There Is No Right Pace for Labor.

If you are birthing in a hospital, it's possible to feel pressure from providers that your labor should be moving at a certain speed.

Policies or pressure around "timing out" or "arrest of progress" (aka being told you need surgery because you've been laboring for a certain amount of time) are based on studies trying to create a standard for a very individualized process. If everyone's health is good and the birther still has the willpower and desire to keep going, it's always okay to ask for more time.

In a similar vein, there is no evidence to support "timing out" from pushing, aka being told you need surgery just because you've been pushing for a certain amount of time. Let us remind you, pushing is hard work. You are literally moving a human being through your pelvis. This should take time! While the recommendation from ACOG is at least two hours of pushing for those who have given birth vaginally before and at least three hours for those who haven't, they also support allowing for more time on an individualized basis.[93] If you're giving birth at home or a birthing center, you likely won't have to worry about the concept of timing out or needing to dilate at a certain speed.

For more tips and tools to stay in the flow of your labor, see pg 213.

WHAT IF . . .
I HAVE BACK LABOR?

Maybe you've heard of "back labor" from friends or people on the interwebs sharing their birth tales. Or maybe this is brand-new information for you. Either way, it is important knowledge to have, so here's a breakdown on what's going on during back labor and some tools to support you.

What Is Back Labor and Why Do You Get It?

Back labor is essentially when you feel strong sensations in your lower back during contractions and sometimes in between them as well. Why? Even if your baby is head down, there can still be variations in their positioning. And this positioning can affect where you feel your contractions, their strength, and the overall course of your labor.

In optimal positioning—meaning baby is able to put the optimal amount of pressure on your cervix to help it open—baby faces *toward* your spine. When you experience back labor, it is often a sign that baby is either facing completely away from your spine, this is called "sunny-side up," "OP," or "posterior presentation"— or that baby's head is cocked slightly toward their shoulder, called asynclitism. In these presentations, baby's head may put extra pressure on the nerves of your spine, causing those intense back labor sensations and sometimes making it more difficult for baby to make it through the birth canal.

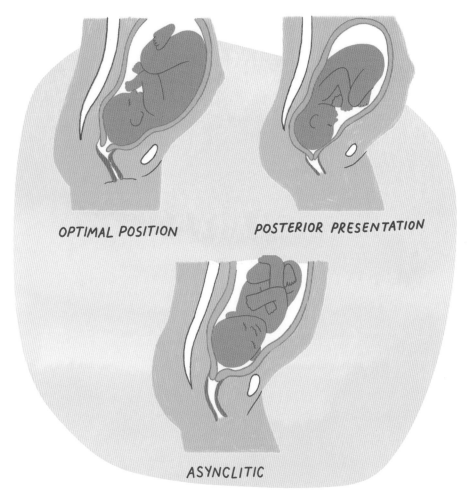

OPTIMAL POSITION   POSTERIOR PRESENTATION

ASYNCLITIC

#BrilliantBIT

Don't stress over baby's position! This is only meant to be a guide so that you can help your body prep and feel like you have tools in case you do find yourself in this situation. It is very common for babies to start off posteriorly or with a cocked head and shift along the way. It is also possible for your baby's head to be tilted or to be facing posteriorly and for you to have no extra discomfort, prolonged labor, or trouble pushing.

WHERE'S YOUR BABY?

While we can't control baby's position, it can be useful—and fun!—for you to start learning how to track what position your baby is in.

- Where in your body do you feel kicks?
- Where do you feel, or not feel, fingers (like a swishy sensation)?
- Where is the butt?

Though baby's position can, and likely will, change over time, it can still be a nice way for you to connect with baby and your body in a new way. As you figure this out, you can also ask your care provider to confirm what you suspect.

While we can't fully control how baby orients inside you, we can try to influence the amount of space in your pelvis so that if baby is able, they can reposition themselves. See pg 218 for tips to create more space in your pelvis during pregnancy.

How Do I Know If My Baby Is in a Nonoptimal Position during Labor?

Aside from searing back discomfort during contractions, if you notice any of the following, it might be an indication that baby's head is tilted or that they are facing sunny-side up:

- Very intense contractions that come every two to three minutes when you're *less than* five or six centimeters dilated.
- You feel lower back pain in between contractions.
- Your contractions are "coupled," meaning they are coming right on top of one another with little break in between.
- You have consistent contractions, but no cervical dilation.
- You feel the "urge to push," but you are not fully dilated.

#BrilliantTIP

If you decide to work with a doula, we recommend you ask them if they feel prepared to help you navigate back labor and if they are able to help detect labor patterns that may indicate a nonoptimal position.

What to Do If You Experience Back Labor

If you start feeling the contractions heavily in your back, it is important to communicate this to your support team so that . . . they can have your back! See pg 216 for tips.

If You're Birthing in a Hospital, Epidurals Can Help!

For some, back labor can be unbearable and the ability to release into the contractions, impossible. An epidural can be useful in these cases to give you a rest from the sensations and allow your body to release. This release may actually be the thing that helps your baby shift positions. If this is what you need, just remember you should still be working to switch positions during labor, helping baby make their way down that canal. See pg 224 for suggestions on how to move with an epi.

WHAT IF . . .
I HAVE A 72-HOUR LABOR?

One of the biggest mindfucks during labor is how to deal with time. Hours can feel like days, or they can feel like minutes. You're likely going to want to know how soon you'll be fully dilated or when you can finally be done. And usually, the answer is *We don't know!*

Very reassuring . . .

While 72-hour labors are possible, they are certainly not the average. But that doesn't mean a 12-, or 24-, or 48-hour labor is necessarily any easier to handle. So how do we deal with this big unknown and not get stuck feeling like it's never going to end?

Let's start by changing our expectations. Unfortunately it is just not true that our water breaks and ten minutes later a fleshy, clean, three-month-old baby slides out. Actually, the average length of labor for first-timers is more like twenty-four hours.[94] Take that in for a second. We know this may sound *impossible*, but, let us explain . . .

The Hardest Part of Contractions Is the Shortest!

Remember, contractions happen in waves. There is a buildup, a peak, a comedown, and then a lull, when those oxytocin receptors fall off, for you to *rest and recover* before the buildup starts happening again. This *rest and recover* time is key! And, as it turns out, it's actually where you spend most of your labor!

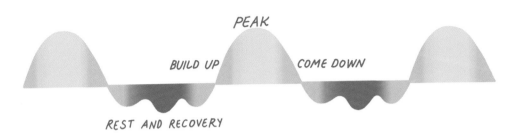

PEAK

BUILD UP   COME DOWN

REST AND RECOVERY

The trick is to take advantage of that downtime. Think about going from *rest period to rest period* instead of from *contraction to contraction*. What this means is that as soon as your contraction starts to comedown, you go back to trying to rest. You may not actually sleep—that's okay!—but at least close your eyes, listen to music, have someone give you a massage, etc. (see more tips on pg 213) and recover by eating some quick fuel, like grapes, and drinking a sip of water. If you're able to give in to truly resting, those rest periods will actually feel longer!

Try This

Imagine you are laying on the beach, just where the ocean hits the sand. It's a beautiful day, the sun is beaming down on your skin, warming you completely. You hear a wave begin and you know that as soon as that water hits your body you will be cold and uncomfortable. You start to brace yourself for the discomfort. You take deep long breaths as the water splashes over you. It sucks. But then, you realize the wave has receded. You start to feel the sunshine on your body again, and you begin to warm up. Instead of focusing on how wet you are, you focus on the sun and its warmth on your skin, and suddenly, you feel dry. You actually feel kind of nice. You hear a wave begin again, and you know you are about to be uncomfortable. But you also know that the discomfort will pass and you'll be able to warm up and get dry again so long as you focus on the sun. This is going *from rest period to rest period!*

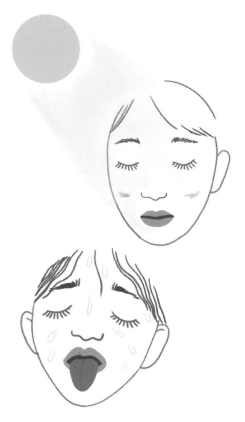

Now imagine you're lying on that beach but you get so afraid of that wave hitting you that your whole body tenses up and you try to escape it. You can't, so you still get soaked, and now you're wet and miserable and you keep moving around trying to avoid the water. And you hear the sound of the wave again, and so you try to escape it again, but you can't, and now you're exhausted from trying to get away from it, and you're still wet and still miserable, and oh no, another wave . . . you get the idea. This is going *from contraction to contraction.*

#BrilliantTIP

If you have an epidural, you hopefully won't be feeling the contractions and will be able to rest more easily—you may even be able to sleep! Sometimes, however, the challenge becomes about passing the time without feeling like you've been laying in bed forever. Check out the Distractions on pg 213.

127

You Don't Contract the Entire Time!

Clinically, labor is often broken down into the following parts (see pg 203 for more on stages of labor). For those who are birthing vaginally for the first time, this will give you a *sense* of what you can expect timing-wise in an unmedicated labor, though there are definitely variations.

EARLY LABOR (until around 5–6 cm)

A couple hours to a couple of days. Contractions have no real pattern at this stage—they can be five minutes apart, twenty minutes apart, eight minutes apart. . . . You'll have the longest *rest and recover* periods between the contractions during this phase.

ACTIVE LABOR (6–8 cm)

Hours, not days. There is a very consistent contraction pattern; generally every three, four, or five minutes. You get shorter and/or fewer *rest and recover* periods in between contractions here, and the contractions feel more intense.

TRANSITION (8–10 cm)

Minutes to hours (but not in the double digits). There is a similar contraction pattern to active labor, though the contractions may last a bit longer and feel more intense. You typically get the least amount of time to *rest and recover* here. But it is also usually the quickest phase.

PUSHING: Minutes to a few hours

For many, the contractions tend to space out once pushing begins. This means more rest time in between pushes to save and build your energy.

BIRTHING THE PLACENTA: Minutes

Once baby is born, the urge to push stops, but your uterus will continue to contract so that the placenta can peel off the uterine wall and you can push it out your vagina. (These won't feel anything like labor contractions). The placenta is usually born between five and forty-five minutes after baby is born.

As you can see, not only is most of *each* contraction spent in downtime, but *most of labor* is spent in the phase where there is the longest period of *rest and recover* between the contractions!

For more tips on how to stay in the flow of long labors and go from rest period to rest period, see pg 213.

Coping with Rest Periods

While there's often lots of emphasis on how to best cope with the contraction sensations, so much about sustaining yourself through labor is actually about how you cope with downtime and how you can truly make it rejuvenating.

Here are some tips to make labor feel shorter by making those rest periods feel better.

GO THE EFF TO SLEEP!

Often labor starts at night, when oxytocin levels tend to naturally peak. Plus, melatonin (a sleep hormone) increases the uterus's sensitivity to oxytocin, which helps get the contractions going. If this happens to you, we can't stress enough the importance of staying in bed and trying to sleep. Resist the urge to call your family, google "what to do with a real live baby?" or start fussing over this and that. And unless you can tell the contractions are coming long, strong, and very consistently without using an app, there's no need to start timing them. Instead, take advantage of the quiet hours to rest up. And if staying in bed is too uncomfortable, try to find a better resting position somewhere else (see pg 223 for recs). We know this is easier said than done, but this is your time to start banking some rest. If you miss out on this period, you're likely going to be much more exhausted later on.

IGNORE IT: IT'S NOT LABOR UNTIL IT'S LABOR.

Until the contractions are strong enough that it's impossible *not* to pay attention to them and they are coming consistently enough that you can't be social in between them, ignore them! If it's daytime and you were able to sleep through the night, try not to psych yourself out that "you're in labor" and instead go about your day—skip the office, though! Move around, eat well, stay hydrated, and pee often. If you were not able to sleep during the night, sleep during the day! And, unless it is obvious without an app that your contractions are coming strong, long, and very consistently, there is *still* no need to time them. There will be a point when it's very clear that those contractions are taking over with a consistent pattern. This is the transition we are looking for and when it makes sense to check in with your app.

#BrilliantBIT

If your labor is heading past twenty-four hours and you have not noticed much change in your contraction pattern, it may be that baby needs some help with their position. See pg 218 for tips on how to create more space for baby to turn.

A NOTE ON PRODROMAL LABOR

Prodromal labor isn't so common, but it is worth mentioning so that you don't feel like a crazy person if it happens to you. Prodromal labor is when you have long, strong contractions, but they don't actually progress into active labor—they just stop at regular intervals. So, for example, you contract all night, but as soon as the sun comes up, the contractions stop entirely. When the sun goes down, they start up again. This can go on for days, even weeks. Prodromal's a bitch, no doubt about it. It's physically and mentally *exhausting* and a really tough hand of cards to be dealt. While the causes are still not entirely clear, it can sometimes be a positional thing, so it is worth trying the suggestions on pg 216. If this happens to you, take advantage of the downtime and sleep during the day, eat nourishing foods, and stay hydrated. Do note that while it is extremely frustrating, often people who experience prodromal labor, have shorter actual labors!

WHAT IF . . .
IT HURTS LIKE HELL?

Because we typically hear only about the pain and horrors of labor—and remember our history!—it's no wonder so many of us can get anxious about what contractions will feel like. But until we experience them, we don't know how they will feel in *our* body. Now we aren't saying the sensations won't be intense, but the discomforts of labor are so often intensified by the Head—our fears, our worries, and our thought patterns.

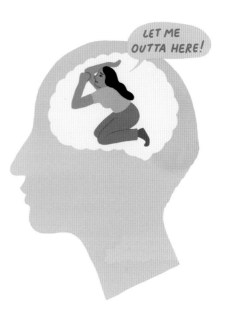

Here are some new ways to change your thinking around contractions and some tools to stay in your Body.

YOU GET PRACTICE.

Nature made contraction patterns pretty smart. While there is always room for variations, for the most part they build up in intensity and duration over time. This means your Body (and Head) have a chance to catch up, get used to how they feel, and produce a ton of hormones that will help you physically cope with the sensations (see pg 75).

CONTRACTIONS DON'T ELICIT A PAIN RESPONSE IN THE BODY.

Again, we aren't saying the sensation won't be incredibly intense, but what you are feeling isn't actually a physiological pain response. When you get injured, your Body typically goes into fight-or-flight and there's an inflammation response to protect it. When you contract, there is an entirely different orchestra of hor-

131

mones at play (remember pg 75!). Also, so much of pain is connected to fear: *Is it broken? Will I ever walk again? Am I out of work for weeks?* In labor, the contraction sensations are a sign things are very right! And the more intense the sensations feel, the closer you are to it being over.

CALL IT WHAT IT IS.

Even though it isn't a *physiological* pain response, there may be times you want to scream during your labor. (Go ahead! Scream it out!) During these times, it is helpful to call out exactly what it is you are feeling, so that you can remember the *productivity* of the sensations and that they are happening *for* you, not *to* you. Generally, a contraction is a mix of three sensations:

- **Tightening and Stretching:** The Uterine Lawnmower! That cervix being lifted up and outta the way so that it can open.
- **Pressure:** Your baby's head is pressing on different parts of your pelvis.

And all three of these sensations are bringing you closer to meeting your baby!

PAIN VS. SUFFERING

Suffering occurs in labor when your Head or Emotions start to take over, you have reached your limit with Body sensations, or you aren't being properly supported. *You should not suffer through your labor.* If at any point you feel like you are, tell your support people so that they can help you and/or advocate for you if needed.

#BrilliantBIT

If you are on Pitocin or experiencing back labor, the severity of the contraction sensations may be more intense and more difficult to override without some help. Be really kind to yourself in these situations and *go inward* to ensure you aren't suffering needlessly.

WHAT ARE *YOUR* GO-TO COPING TECHNIQUES?

Before you go into labor, exploring your personal relationship to discomfort and fear can be a powerful exercise. We all have our own tricks and tools we've picked up over the years that may actually be useful in labor too.

Think back to times you have been physically uncomfortable, afraid, or anxious:

- What did your Head do? Did it race? Did it go blank?
- What did your Body do? Did your shoulders tense? Jaw clench? Did you hold your breath? Close your eyes?
- What coping techniques did your Gut tell you to use to get through the experience? Meditate? Watch TV? Take medicine?
- Who helped you?

Learning how you've responded to discomfort and fear in the past can give you lots of information and tools that can help you get through your labor! You may want to write a few of your answers down to share with your support team.

See pg 213 for more tips and tools for coping through your labor and remember to Go Inward (see pg 100) to see if it's your Body or your Head causing the discomfort!

WHAT IF . . .
I HAVE TO TRANSFER?

If you are planning to give birth at home or at a birth center, transferring to a hospital may be the last thing you want to think about. But thinking through your transfer plan doesn't mean you will have to do it! It's just that it is impossible to plan your birth, so staying open to the possibility of needing access to medication, surgical procedures, or simply a change of scenery, along with feeling confident in how the transfer will go down if it does become necessary, can actually *help you* stay in the flow of your labor, while also being superuseful if you need to go with your Plan B.

TRANSFERS ARE RARE AND USUALLY NOT AN EMERGENCY.

Hopefully you already have a sense of your midwife's transfer rate and most common reasons for transfers. You'll likely hear that most of the time the transfer is not an emergency—meaning the pregnant person gets too tired, decides they want or need an epidural, or the labor or pushing phase has been extremely long. Actual emergency situations are rare, but it's helpful to ask your midwife for a breakdown of how many of their transfers were true emergencies.

TALKING TO YOUR MIDWIFE ABOUT YOUR TRANSFER PLAN.

Your provider should lead the discussion on what will go down if a transfer does become necessary, but here are some questions you can ask to guide the conversation.

- What are the most common scenarios for transfer?
- Where would we transfer to if it is an emergency? Where would we transfer to if it's not an emergency?
- Do you have relationships with the doctors/midwives at these hospitals?

- What is the transfer process like in a nonemergency situation? In a emergency situation?

- What is the transfer process like if it is for an issue that arises during labor vs. postpartum?

- If I'm the one transferring (as opposed to the baby needing to be transferred), will you stay with me in the hospital?

- What happens if it is the baby that needs medical attention? Can you walk me through how this goes down?

- What happens once the baby or I am discharged from the hospital? Will I come back into your care for postpartum visits?

GET TO KNOW THE HOSPITAL.

This is an important step so that you can really understand what to expect in case a transfer is necessary. Some things to consider:

- Which is the closest hospital vs. which is your ideal hospital? You'll go to the closest in case of an emergency, but otherwise you'll probably want to go where you'll feel the most comfortable—because that's where your midwife has relationships, because they have a reputation of being more open to transfers, or because you know the postpartum care is best.

- Get to know the hospital(s)' policies. Do they routinely separate parents from babies? Are partners allowed to stay postpartum? Are they friendly to transfers? Many hospitals offer tours—this may be something to consider to get all your questions answered in advance.

- Pack a bag. In the rare case you need to run out the door, it might be nice to have some things all ready to bring with you. Don't go crazy here: just bring the essentials, as someone can always go back home to get you the rest of your stuff. You may also want to consider bringing some vibes to make you feel more at home once there.

WHAT IF . . .
THE "CASCADE OF INTERVENTIONS" HAPPENS TO ME?

An intervention is an action taken by your provider that quite literally "intervenes" with the physiological labor process. The "cascade of interventions" is the idea that once one intervention is introduced, another will be introduced, and then another, and another until a cesarean is needed.

The root of the fear here is twofold:

1 You're going to lose all control of your labor.

2 You end up having a cesarean birth (for those who really wanted a vaginal birth).

In some circles, interventions have gotten a bad rap because they are overused and often administered without real informed consent. But just as it is important to recognize that interventions may be overused, it is also important to realize they can be major lifesavers and sometimes just the trick to move you through your labor.

While there are many different interventions, the most common are IVs, continuous monitoring devices, induction and augmentation medications (like Pitocin), artificially rupturing the membranes (i.e., your practitioner breaks your water), epidurals, assisted delivery instruments (forceps or vacuum), and surgery (C-section).

Two Ways to Think about Interventions

1 **Interventions you know you want:** If you are someone who is considering an elective surgery or induction or is entering their birth knowing they want an epidural, it's important to

136

take the time to understand the risks and benefits of these procedures, as well as learn how exactly they go down. This will help you decide if it truly is the best option for you and your baby and, if so, prepare you for what to expect.

2 **Interventions you only want if necessary:** Even if you are birthing at home, the potential for interventions still exists. We find it helpful to shift your thinking away from "interventions I want to avoid" and instead lean into "interventions I'm open to having *if* they become necessary."

The Truth about Interventions

MANY INTERVENTIONS COME WITH OTHER INTERVENTIONS.

It's important to understand that most interventions come in "packages." This means if you get one, you will likely need others. For example, if you opt for an epidural, you'll also get an IV, continuous monitoring, a pulsometer, a blood pressure cuff, and a bladder catheter since you won't be able to get up to pee.

While this is to ensure everyone's safety, in the moment it can feel like you've suddenly become E.T. Understanding ahead of time that you are signing up for "packages" can help you adjust your expectations—though unfortunately, there's nothing we can do about all of those wires! However, if an intervention is introduced, it doesn't mean you will definitely need surgery or lose your ability to play an active role in your care!

#BrilliantTIP

A good question to ask the care provider before agreeing to an intervention is "What else does this intervention come with?"

INTERVENTIONS DON'T ALWAYS *LEAD* TO OTHER INTERVENTIONS, BUT THEY DO *INCREASE YOUR CHANCES* OF NEEDING THEM.

Just because you introduce one intervention, doesn't mean that you will need others. But it is helpful to stay open to them, as each intervention does up your chances of needing another one. For instance, getting an epidural doesn't mean that you will have a C-section, but it can increase your chances of needing one if your labor is not active yet.[95] Getting Pitocin doesn't mean that you'll need an epidural, but it does increase your chances of needing one. Getting an epidural doesn't mean you'll need Pitocin, but it does increase your chances of needing it.[96] You get the picture.

INTERVENTIONS CAN ACTUALLY *HELP YOU* AVOID A C-SECTION.

We've seen plenty of people have vaginal births even with all the interventions. In fact, sometimes it is exactly those interventions that allow for a healthy vaginal birth to take place. This is why it is so important to *go inward* throughout labor (see pg 100). When you are making decisions from your Body and Gut and not your (or your practitioner's) fears throughout your labor, you are going to know what you need. And if you truly trust you need the intervention, then you are always making the right decision!

Avoiding Unnecessary Interventions

STAY HOME AS LONG AS YOU CAN.

If you are birthing in a hospital and have no medical issues that necessitate otherwise, labor at home for as long as possible. The longer you are in the hospital, the more susceptible you are to interventions.

It's probably too soon to go to the hospital if:

- You can still talk through contractions.
- You can sit down and have a meal.
- You can post on social media or call your friends and family.
- You can get to the car without needing to stop for contractions on your way.

This being said, if at any point your Gut tells you it's time to go, then it's definitely time to go!

#LaborTOOL

No matter where you're birthing and with whom, there might be times during labor when something comes up and you'll have to make a decision on how to move forward. These moments can be overwhelming and bring up feelings of frustration, fear, exhaustion, and even mistrust in your Body. It may feel like you no longer know what you want or need, or what's best for you, yet you need to give an answer ASAP. The truth is that real emergencies are rare and you will know if you are in the middle of one. Otherwise, there's generally time, and it's important for you to take it. Use this tool:

B.R.A.N.D.*

This easy acronym reminds you how to navigate the conversation when an intervention is being recommended.

B = What are the **Benefits?**

R = What are the **Risks?**

A = What are the **Alternatives?**

N = What happens if we do **Nothing?**

D = Do we have time to **Decide?**

This is not a Nat + Ash original. It's been floating around in the doula community, and we don't know who created it originally!

Remaining an Active Participant in Your Labor

THE PATIENT-CENTERED WAY FOR INTERVENTIONS TO BE USED

1   An intervention is recommended because the pregnant person is asking for it or because of the pregnant person's unique and particular labor—not simply because of policies or protocols.

2   The pregnant person's Body or Gut is telling them that the intervention is truly functioning as a tool for their and/or baby's safety or ability to keep going.

3   The pregnant person—or their medical proxy—understands the full risks and benefits of the intervention and consents to its use *prior* to it being administered. This goes for *all* interventions—even those that come in "packages" or are needed because of previous interventions introduced.

Here is where we remind you that it is not about *the path*. It is about how you *move through it*. You are not less capable because you need Pitocin, opt for an epidural, or end up with a cesarean birth. The most awesome skill of labor is being able to *go inward* (see pg 100) and trust what you *really* need along the way.

Here's one more tool to help you do that.

WHAT IF . . .
I'M TOLD I NEED A C-SECTION?

Let us start by saying there is nothing wrong with cesareans. For some, it's the safest way to have a baby. It is our right as pregnant people to have a say in how our babies are born, including having a cesarean birth. Still, you must understand the risks and benefits for your individual situation (*individual decision-making* time!) to know if a cesarean is *actually* the safest choice for you.

Here's the lowdown.

Planned Cesareans vs. "Emergency" Cesareans

Planned cesarean births are surgeries that are decided on ahead of time—it's when a date is put on the books for you to meet your baby. All surgery births that are not "on the books" are lumped under the category "emergency C-section." This means that most of those "emergency C-sections" you hear about are actually just *unplanned* C-sections. Very few are true emergencies!

Planned Cesareans

Some reasons why a C-section may be planned:

○ The birthing person has preexisting medical conditions.

○ The placenta is covering the cervix.

○ There are concerns about baby's health.

○ It's safest for the mental and emotional health of the birthing person.

○ Baby is not head down. (Unfortunately, there's a very limited number of care providers with the expertise to support vaginal breech births, so in the United States most are born via surgery.) If your baby is in a transverse lie (chilling horizontally in your uterus), a C-section will also be needed.

○ The birthing person elects it.

And then, there are the common reasons not always supported by medical evidence—and likely contributing to our high cesarean rates in America:

○ **You had a C-section for your last birth.** Even though the current research indicates that it is safer to attempt a vaginal birth after cesarean (VBAC) than to have another surgery,[97] it can be difficult to find a care provider willing to support you in this decision.

○ **You are carrying multiples.** Current research does not support C-section for twin pregnancies where at least one of the babies is head down.[98] However, many practitioners recommend C-sections for twins anyway, and most professional organizations recommend cesarean birth if you're having three or more babies.

○ **Your baby is measuring big.** You already know this one! See pg 105 for more.

142

True Emergencies vs. Unplanned Cesarean Births

TRUE EMERGENCIES

In the rare case of a true emergency, things will likely start to move very quickly. Your provider will explain what is going on, but there may not be much time for questions. That being said, you, or your medical proxy, will still need to consent to the surgery. This is why trusting your care provider is important—so that if there is a true emergency, you feel taken care of and don't have to question the validity of the emergency.

UNPLANNED CESAREAN BIRTHS

Most of the time though, there is plenty of time to talk it all through, and in some cases, your provider will have already planted the seed that surgery might be necessary earlier in your labor to give you more time to process. Remember to go inward (see pg 100) and use B.R.A.N.D. (see pg 139).

WAYS TO REDUCE YOUR RISK OF AN UNPLANNED SURGERY

- Find a care provider with low cesarean rates. If you are low-risk, don't work with a practice that specializes in high-risk pregnancies.
- Stay home until your labor is very active.
- Move around during labor and ask for intermittent monitoring instead of continuous monitoring (see below).
- Stay upright as much as possible before pushing, or move through different laying positions if you have an epidural (see pg 224).
- Work with a doula.
- Exercise during pregnancy.[99]

#BrilliantBIT

Despite being commonly used in hospitals, continuous electronic fetal monitoring is *not* supported by clinical evidence for those who are low-risk and have no interventions. In fact, all professional organizations, including ACOG,[100] AWHONN, and ACNM,[101] recommend intermittent monitoring as the standard of practice for all low-risk pregnancies. Not only does continuous electronic fetal monitoring *not* reduce perinatal mortality, but it ends up increasing your risk of having an unnecessary C-section[102] and of having an assisted delivery (both vacuum and forceps[103]).

#BrilliantBIT

True intermittent monitoring, as recommended by ACOG, is listening to the baby's heart with a handheld wireless monitor for 1 minute every 15–30 minutes during active labor, and 1 minute every 5–15 minutes during pushing.[104] It doesn't mean being on the electronic monitor for 20 minutes every hour like we see in many hospital settings. Ask about your options!

Talk It Through before Labor.

For those really wanting to avoid surgery, we understand the inclination to skip knowing any details about how the procedure might go down. But cesareans are major abdominal surgery and understanding some of the process ahead of time can make the experience less traumatic. Sometimes, by letting our fears in, we end up letting them go. Remember that talking about it doesn't mean it is going to happen to you.

Regardless of whether you are planning surgery or not, it's a good idea to have your care provider, doula, or childbirth educator walk you through the process at your particular hospital and answer the following questions:

- What are the risks?
- What type of uterine closure will be used—single or double layer? Would it be strong enough to support another labor (especially important if you plan on having more children and want to attempt a VBAC).
- How many support people are allowed to be in the OR?
- Would my partner or support team and I be separated at any points before or after the surgery?
- How long would it take?
- What physical sensations would there be during surgery?
- How soon after the surgery would I be able to be with my baby?
- How long would I need to stay at the hospital after?
- What would I expect to feel immediately after surgery and in the days/weeks that follow?

There are also things you can request to make the experience feel gentler—also called gentle cesarean. After you get an idea of what the process looks like, you can go through the following preferences:

- Could we play music during the surgery?
- Could I watch the baby be born? (Don't worry, you won't see your insides or anything! The drape can be lowered so that you can just see babe come out, Simba style. It may not be your cup of tea, but if this piques your interest, ask!)
- Could I do some skin-to-skin with my baby in the OR?

A warning for partners: Because you typically enter the OR after the birthing person has already been set up, it can be a bit shocking and overwhelming to see your loved one laid out on an operating table. Take some deep breaths before you go in, and if you need to step out at any point throughout the surgery, that's okay! Better to take a break than pass out.

> **#BrilliantBIT**
>
> **A note on vaginal seeding:** We'll add this here since some of you may have heard of it. . . . *Seeding* is a much more pleasant way of saying "taking a swab of vaginal fluids and smearing it all over my baby." Why do that? The idea is that because babies born via cesarean are introduced to the hospital's bacteria before their parent's bacteria, "seeding" will allow baby to make use of your beneficial bacteria. It is important to note that ACOG *does not* recommend this practice because of the risk of passing an infection on to baby. And at the time of writing, there is no research supporting the benefits of this practice. This being said, things are always changing so if this piques your interest, you can always talk with your care provider.

WHAT IF . . .
I POOP MYSELF WHILE PUSHING?

Here's the thing—you just may.

In fact, that infamous "urge to push" sensation is actually somewhat akin to the sensation of really, *really* needing to poop. Take a moment to revisit where the pelvic outlet is on your body (pg 219). Yeah . . . that's the cause of that sensation—turns out, you have a butt full of baby!

> **#BrilliantTIP**
>
> In your final weeks of pregnancy we encourage you to start paying attention to your body when you go to the bathroom. What muscles do you use to poop? What is your face doing—is it all scrunched up and tense? Are your shoulders to your ears? Can you practice releasing those parts and putting all your effort into your push? Of course, this isn't exactly the same as pushing a baby out, but we do find this can be great practice nonetheless.

While we totally get that the idea of pooping in front of people is a turnoff, we encourage you to push past it! (Literally!) Squeezing that baby through the birth canal takes effort—so we need you at 100 percent. Plus, if you poop while you push, it's actually a good sign that you are pushing with the right muscles.

It may also make you feel better to know that generally, it's not a full-on poop sesh—most people will release just a little bit, we promise! So much is going on, you probably won't even know it happened and the nurse or birth assistant will clean it up superfast.

#BrilliantTIP
Thanks to those prostaglandins, many people have a good "clean out" during early labor or prior to starting labor (hello, diarrhea!). Either way, remember to go to the bathroom throughout labor to continue emptying out and creating more space for baby. (You'll want to keep your bladder empty too.)

#BrilliantTIP
Have some fresh-smelling essential oils on hand during pushing. We like using eucalyptus, mint, or lemon. Aside from the poop, sometimes there can be some strong smells during the pushing phase, so taking a whiff in between pushes is a great way to refresh and reenergize.

WHAT IF . . .
MY VAGINA TEARS OPEN?

Just reading that makes most of us cringe! Vaginal changes from childbirth are real, but they don't need to be so scary—while tearing rates are variable and depend on the birthing person's body, birth setting, and care provider practices, 53–79 percent of people will have some type of laceration at vaginal delivery,[105] so it's time we start normalizing it, because if you tear, it doesn't mean you did anything wrong. Stick with us.

What Is a Tear and Why Does It Happen?

As baby's head comes out and the perineum stretches, sometimes the pressure is a bit too much and can cause injuries to the skin, muscles, or in rare cases, the tissues. There are different degrees of tearing.

THE MOST COMMON

FIRST DEGREE: When there are lacerations to the skin and mucosa layer. This is the most superficial type of tear and is the quickest to heal. They rarely even needs stitches! This can happen on the labia, vagina, or perineal area.

SECOND DEGREE: When the muscle layer is also involved in the tear. This is the most common type of tear and typically requires stitches to repair.

THE LEAST COMMON

THIRD DEGREE: When the tear involves the internal and/or external anal sphincter.

FOURTH DEGREE: When the tear also involves the rectum and the tissues that surround it. This is the severest type of tearing (and least common) and requires a skilled provider that can do a surgical repair.

SOME OTHER POSSIBILITIES

- **Superficial lacerations on the labia.** These "skid marks" usually don't require stitches but can make it sting a little—or a lot—when you pee. It's not ideal, we know, but these tend to heal quickly.

- **No tearing or lacerations at all!** Often, home birth and birth center–based midwives have lower rates of tears, but it is definitely also possible to come out of a hospital birth without lacerations.

Minimizing Your Risk of Tearing

IN PREGNANCY

PERINEAL MASSAGE. Massaging your perineum during the last weeks of pregnancy can help you get familiar with how it feels when your perineum stretches and when pressure is applied (you might need a partner's help if you can't reach all the way down there!). While there isn't much research to support or disprove this, we do hear experientially that it helps, and if nothing else, it's a good practice to help you get used to the sensations of that area stretching, since it's so foreign for most of us! Warning: this doesn't feel *good*. So be sure to go slow and check in along the way. If you have experienced sexual trauma, this sensation may be triggering, so be extra communicative. We recommend using some kind of lube or oil to keep things movin' and, while you're at it, you might as well try to have some fun with it if you can! See the resources on pg 249 to learn how to perform this massage.

EAT COLORFUL, NUTRIENT-RICH, WHOLE FOODS AND FATS. This may seem obvious, but getting those antioxidants, particularly vitamin C, is vital to tissue health and resilience. Be sure to get those healthy fats too—from foods like avocado, organic eggs, nuts, grass-fed organic meats, etc.

AS YOU PUSH

SELF-DIRECT. Particularly if you are birthing with an OB in a hospital, the tendency is for them to coach you to hold your breath as you push and they count to 10. The most vagina-friendly way to push is to go with your Body's cues and not hold your breath. Even if you need some direction to get the party started, going with your impulses from there will reduce the impact on your perineum. While this can be more difficult if you have an epidural, it is still possible to feel that pressure!

GO SLOW. If you don't have an epidural, as your baby's head crowns and your perineal tissues and muscles stretch, you might start feeling a burning sensation like no other (often called the ring of fire, see pg 210). You may be tempted to scream and not give a hoot about anything other than getting that baby out. But if you can, try to slow it down. While the ring of fire may not be as intense for those with epidurals, the same rule still applies. Most likely at this point your provider will guide you as to when to let your body push *for you* (remember that giant fundus pressing on baby!) versus when you need to give some extra oomph. We know it's hard, but if you can refrain from actively pushing at this point, you will minimize your risk of tearing, as this allows for the baby's head to stretch the tissues over time.

AVOID PUSHING ONLY ON YOUR BACK. People who give birth on all fours are the least likely to experience genital tract trauma. Pushing on your side is another good option. Laying on your back, squatting, or the standard pelvic exam position (laying on your back with your feet up on stirrups) can increase the risk of tearing.[106] If you have an epidural, you should still be able to move from side to side and maybe even get on all fours to push—just ask your team for help if your legs feel heavy.

WARM COMPRESS. One of the best approaches to reducing deep tearing during pushing is to have your care provider press a warm compress against your perineum as you push.[107] If you think there's a chance you might want this, make sure to let your care provider know ahead of time. Remember, you can always ask them to stop.

MASSAGE. To help you stretch as you push, some providers do perineal massage with oil. A review of a number of studies[108] suggests that massage can minimize the risk of third- and fourth-degree tears. However, for some people this can be painful, triggering, and/or very uncomfortable, so make sure to speak up if you don't want anyone's hands down there. You can always change your mind and switch it up later as well; start with massage and then ask them to stop or vice versa.

WATER BIRTH. If you give birth in the water, you are less likely to have third- or fourth-degree tears.[109] Also, if you want to be left alone, pushing in the water makes it more difficult for anyone to touch your perineum or baby, other than yourself! Unfortunately though, many hospitals don't allow water births, so do your research on your birthing location if this is a route you're interested in.

Episiotomies vs. Tearing

An episiotomy is when the perineal area is intentionally cut by a care provider. (Eek!) Until somewhat recently, episiotomies accompanied most vaginal births, as medical professionals believed it was safer than letting the perineal area tear on its own. Lucky for us, nowadays we know that an episiotomy does not actually prevent a tear from happening and can actually *increase* the chance of having a third- or fourth-degree tear.[110] Episiotomies are no longer recommended unless an instrumental birth (vacuum or forceps) is needed—and not in all cases!—or if baby needs to be born very quickly in an emergency situation. Otherwise, a natural tear is less painful and heals more quickly.[111] Plus, without an episiotomy there is also the chance that you won't tear at all.

> **#BrilliantTIP**
> While episiotomies aren't so routine anymore, they are still done and often can be done without you even knowing it is happening. Be sure to let your provider know that you would like to consent to the cut *before* it happens.

Healing

The healing process is a bit different for every body and dependent upon the severity of the injury. But, overall, your perineum and vagina were built to stretch and are quite resilient. Tearing is very, very normal and not an indication that you did anything wrong. Sometimes, it just happens—even if you went slow, even if you did perineal massage every night, even if you ate all those oranges. For most people that have first- and second-degree tears there is some discomfort during the first couple of weeks postpartum, and then things start to feel better pretty quickly. If you got stitches, they will likely fall out on their own. If you have a deeper tear, you may be given pain medication, and you will likely need to follow up with your provider. Be sure to have a conversation with your provider about your specific perineal care needs after your baby is born. And, regardless of the severity of your injuries, we always recommend seeing a PT or pelvic floor specialist (see more on pg 201).

Want some tips on how to soothe your perineal area in the postpartum period? See pg 232.

WHAT IF . . .
SOMETHING GOES WRONG?

Oh, the ultimate fear. It's almost impossible *not* to think about the worst-case scenarios, particularly if you've had a long journey conceiving or a history of loss. The idea here isn't to ignore these thoughts or push them aside, because they are real. Let's just pause to acknowledge these feelings are there, they are normal, and they are totally okay to have. Almost all pregnant people have them.

The following are some tools that may be useful to prevent these thoughts from overpowering you or getting in the way of your birth.

MAKE SURE YOU TRUST YOUR PROVIDER. If you've gotten this far into the book, you know how important it is that your care provider is a good match for you. You have to be able to trust them! It will make such a big difference in how safe you feel throughout this entire process. If you're not quite there yet, remember there may still be time to switch providers—and it may be worth the effort!

STEP AWAY FROM THAT COMPUTER. If something feels off or you have a question or concern, it's always best to call your provider for medical concerns or check in with your doula instead of asking Google. As you likely already know, it is easy to spiral out when you resort to the deep, dark web.

TAKE CARE OF YOUR EMOTIONS AND BODY. Building your squad is vital here. See pg 199 for more info.

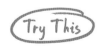

GROUNDING DOWN

When we get stuck in the fear of something going wrong, it can be hard to *drop in* (see pg 20) and connect with our babies, since our Bodies or our babies may be the ones triggering the fear. So if you need another way to ground yourself when you feel like your Head or Emotions are taking over, try these things:

- Mindfulness techniques like visualizations or meditations
- Doing housework or organizing your physical space
- Baking or cooking
- Going on a walk
- Doing a prenatal yoga flow
- Getting into nature
- Hanging with animals

A NOTE ON PREGNANCY AFTER LOSS

Navigating pregnancy after a loss can be especially hard. Because you've already experienced so much pain, the thought of surviving another trauma may feel impossible. You may be hesitant to bond with the baby out of fear of what might happen if you do. You may also feel afraid, guilty, or like it's unjust to experience any joy around this pregnancy. This is all totally normal; it's your defense mechanism against heartbreak. Know this: it's okay to feel all these things. Getting support and talking with other people that have experienced loss and gone on to have another baby may be helpful. It's possible that this pregnancy might actually be an opportunity for you to process some unreleased Emotions of what happened before and transform some of your *blocks*.

part

4

THE
POSTPARTUM
WHAT-IFS

NOW THAT WE'VE SPENT LOTS OF TIME PREPPING FOR LABOR, WE KNOW you're probably starting to wonder about your postpartum self. *Who are you going to become? How are you going to keep that baby alive? How's your body going to feel? What about your relationships? Your work?* We're so glad you asked!

In this section we'll dive into some of those postpartum what-ifs to better prepare you for what's ahead and clear some of those misconceptions.

The early weeks postpartum are times of *big transitions* and come with profound emotional, physical, and mental challenges. This is typically some of the most unwieldy forest you'll trek through. As you read through this section, know that no matter how your postpartum journey looks, you will make it through! And you're going to learn so much along the way.

You've got this.

WHAT IF . . .
I CAN'T STAND MY IN-LAWS?

For some, bringing friends and family into your labor and postpartum experience—IRL and virtually—is exciting. For others, it can be very stressful. We've found that setting boundaries and expectations ahead of time is key.

Here are some suave ways to do so.

During Labor

DECIDE *WHEN* TO TELL PEOPLE YOU'RE IN LABOR.

The moment you tell your peeps you are in labor, they are likely going to be blowing up your phone until baby is born. And then there are those pesky in-laws—and parents!—that show up to your birthing place uninvited. If none of this sounds like your cup of tea, a nice way to avoid it is to hold off on telling people that you're in labor. Remember, it can still be days before your baby is actually born. And for those birthing in a hospital, many only allow two visitors in the labor room at a time. When to share is totally a personal choice, but give yourself permission to wait if you think sharing can become a source of stress.

#BrilliantTIP

For those who want to include others in their labor but don't want to be attached to their phones—and aren't worried about unwanted visitors showing up—a nice way to bring people in is to have them light candles when you first go into labor. This way you both know you are thinking about one another, and the expectation has already been set that you will not be checking in or giving updates throughout.

Postpartum

SHARE YOUR "VISITING SCHEDULE" AHEAD OF TIME.

Unless you are having a planned surgery, it will be impossible to actually make a schedule, but you can let people know ahead of time what *type* of visiting schedule you will have: *only on Tuesdays, only in the afternoons, none on weekends, only for two hours at a time.* This way no one feels singled out, and everyone knows what to expect.

#BrilliantTIP

If you think you won't want others to hold the baby, it is also a good idea to share this in advance. "We prefer to be the only ones handling the baby for the first few weeks. Just wanted to give you a heads-up!"

#BrilliantTIP

Is someone overstaying their welcome? Use breast/chest-feeding as an excuse for privacy or an escape.

DO. NOT. PLAY. HOST.

We can't stress this enough. The people you allow over need to be there to take care of you, not the other way around. We highly recommend giving out tasks to those who won't be helpful on their own. Ask them to take out the trash, pick up some groceries, go to the pharmacy, do your laundry, get you food, feed the cat, etc. Usually the people in your life actually *want* to help, they just don't know how. By giving them specific tasks, you are actually making it easier for them.

WHAT IF . . .
I LOSE MYSELF?

Becoming a parent is wild. It's one of the most dramatic, life-altering experiences a human can have . . . and you can hear that a million times, yet when it actually happens to you, it will *still* blow your mind. Once that baby is placed on your lap, everything changes—your sense of time, how you relate to the world, your body . . . even your brain changes![112]

And yet you will still be *you*.

So how do you hold all these things at once?

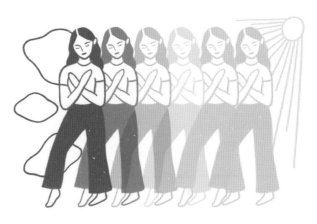

Mourn the Loss.

As you create space in your life for this little babe, it may feel like you are giving up so much of what you felt made you, *you*. There are going to be parts that seem easy—you probably won't miss waking up hungover on a Saturday—but there are also parts that are going to be really hard to let go of. And this might make you feel a little claustrophobic and crazy at times. It's important to acknowledge that, as excited as you may be to meet your little one, there is also a loss here.

Let yourself feel that.

Over time, you're likely to fill those holes with the wonders of your parenthood journey—even if there are parts of it that always kind of suck. Eventually parenthood may actually begin to feel more like an expansion of yourself than a restriction. You'll find yourself being more efficient with your time, prioritizing what's really important in your life, cutting out the BS, laughing and singing more often. Parenthood requires such strength—you may be surprised by how proud of yourself you become. Really!

Some Physical and Emotional Humps to Get Over

"BOUNCE BACK" MY ASS!

For almost ten whole months your body grew and shifted, created new parts, and worked a double shift to accommodate your babe. So it seems unfair to expect for it to "bounce back" quickly to its pre-pregnancy self. Here's the truth: Your body *will* change. You might eventually lose those extra pounds, but it will probably still *feel* different. It won't be the way it was. *It can't* be the way it was because *you grew and birthed a baby!* That's like saying you want the same body you had when you were fifteen. See if you can allow your body changes to be representative of your new superpowers.

TOUCHED-OUT

Particularly if you are breast/chest-feeding, you may start to feel like your body doesn't belong to you anymore. And, even if you aren't breast/chest-feeding, babies want to be held 24/7, so feelings of resentment and ickiness—and then guilt for feeling those feelings!—may still arise. It's very normal to experience this, and it's totally cool to not want to be a human pacifier.

Sometimes, these feelings of being *touched-out* may bleed into your relationship. This can be hard if your partner is feeling like they aren't getting *enough* touch from you. Try to help your partner understand, as it is likely difficult for them to *get it* because they aren't *in it* in quite the same way. (Partners, take note! See pg 240.) You might find that prioritizing alone time is essential. Taking those five minutes to yourself whenever you can, can go a long way. . . . Keep reading for suggestions.

IS THIS THING ON? BRAIN CHANGES.

Lots of people experience "new-parent brain": having a hard time focusing or returning a work email, forgetting what you needed to order from Amazon, etc. And while it might be a little annoying at times, it turns out you're actually just getting smarter at caring for your kid! New research tells us that pregnancy and childbirth do in fact change our brains[113] to enhance our abilities to bond with our babies and recognize social threats. Those changes are actually preparing us for parenthood!

CAN I RETURN THE BABY?

Sometimes you may feel like you want to run away and never come back. And other times, you'll find yourself never wanting to leave your babe's side. We're used to thinking things need to be one way or the other, but they rarely are. Our flaring contradictory emotions are what make us humans so incredibly rich and interesting. See what happens when you embrace it all!

I WANT A DIVORCE.

It's important to remember that your partner is also having an experience, but one that is different from yours. It has to be different than yours because they are not going through the physicality of the postpartum period, and so it may be hard for them to fully understand and empathize with you. And while your partner may not always be able to verbalize this, they too are also going through new feelings—new stressors from identity shifts, new financial pressures, less attention from you, feelings of inadequacy because they don't know how to support you. They may not always be able to give you exactly what you need. We know this can be frustrating, and you may find yourself feeling like your partner doesn't care or isn't supportive. Try to tap into their experience. This doesn't mean sacrificing your needs; it just means to try and give them the benefit of the doubt. They can't read your mind, so ask for what you need.

Do Not Sacrifice Your Own Care.

Most new parents will agree that it can feel almost impossible to find time for some self-care—and when you do, Netflix suddenly feels *way* more appealing than a yoga class. But we can't stress enough the importance of finding some *you* time. Your sanity *is* your baby's health. The better you take care of *you,* the better you'll be able to take care of baby.

Here are some suggestions to help you feel more like a human and less like a feeding machine:

- Go outside each day, even if it's just for a couple of minutes, to take a few deep breaths or go on a walk if you can.

- Have at least one conversation each day about non-baby-related things.

- Blast your fave playlist while you're in the shower.

- Splurge on that sitter every once in a while—or do a trade with someone!

- Ask for help. Really. You can't do it all on your own. At least not all the time. Call your squad (see pg 199).

- Create rituals around your feedings so that as you are feeding baby, you are also feeding yourself. Call a friend. Eat something delicious. Watch your favorite show, or listen to a podcast. Treat yourself!

WHAT IF . . .
I END UP WITH A SAGGY CHEST, A POOCH, AND A STRETCHED-OUT VAG FOREVER?

Oh boy, are we familiar with this worry. How can we not be when the Kardashians' flawless post-baby bodies stare at us from the magazine rack? Not to mention the fact that doctors used to perform procedures called "husband stitches" in which they, no joke, gave patients some extra perineal stitching after episiotomies so that they were "tighter" for their husbands post-birth.

Thankfully, we are coming around to the fact that these examples are representations of the darker side of our culture and not indicative of how birth—or the body—actually works!

But with that said, it *is* true that your parts *do* change in order to accommodate your babe. And even though our bodies are really good at healing themselves, that doesn't mean they don't need support in order to optimally do so. The cool thing is we've found that the more we can build a supportive relationship with our bodies along the way, the better our relationship to them will be later on. Here's how you can start giving some TLC to those more sensitive parts!

Meet Your New Breasts/Chest.

Even if you decide not to breast/chest-feed, you may find that your chest is *way* bigger than it was pre-pregnancy thanks to the expansion of all those milk ducts. While some people's breasts/chest may return to pre-pregnancy size/ shape, many do not, as the flow of milk can permanently stretch your breast/ chest skin and tissues. (Hello, stretch marks!) The reality is, as we age, our chests start pointing south whether we've birthed or not—we might as well just thank them for their service!

In your pregnancy you can start by:

- Staying superhydrated and eat nutrient-rich foods with healthy fats. This will help your tissues and skin stretch with more ease and, sometimes, less visibility.

- Regularly giving yourself gentle breast/chest massages with coconut oil, cocoa butter, or a stretch-mark reduction cream (make sure the one you choose is safe for baby postpartum). Remember to start from your armpits as you have ducts there too!

See pg 228 for tips on taking care of them while breast/chest-feeding.

You Can't Actually Stretch Out Your Vagina!

Many people have a misconception that the vagina is like a giant gaping hole or tube that can have a bigger or smaller diameter. The truth is that the vaginal walls touch one another—meaning that anything that passes through is asking those walls to part. As a result, it's kind of a tight squeeze no matter what.

Even so, the vagina is elastic and made of muscles, and muscles sometimes need some help so that they don't get too tight or too weak, particularly after they just had a *major* workout. Remember, these muscles are connected to your pelvic floor, which is connected to your perineum, anus, and core (the gang's all here!). So taking care of the whole fam, not just individual parts, is important since they can all affect each other, especially postpartum!

During pregnancy, perineal massage and deep abdominal breathing are a great way to start loving on that area and getting yourself acquainted with your pelvic floor (see pg 86).

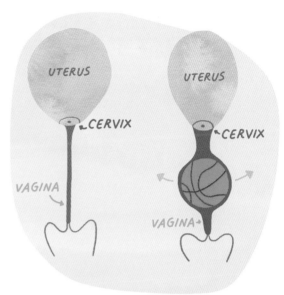

Postpartum, once your stitches come out and you get the go-ahead from your practitioner, continuing with massage at the site can help break up any adhesions as well as build up your readiness to be intimate again.

TAP INTO YOUR NEW CORE STRENGTH.

Remember, your core is connected to your vagina via the pelvic floor. Just as you are tapping into your *core strength* as a new parent, it's important to tend to your, er, *core* strength. Because it takes time for the uterus to return to its previous size and location and your abdominal muscles have been loosened in the process, you may still look pregnant for some time even after you have given birth. (Sorry!) If you have a "pooch" that just won't go away, it can be a clue that some ab separation has occurred. About two-thirds of those who give birth have some abdominal muscle separation post-birth (called diastasis recti). This can get better on its own with time, but depending on the severity of the separation, it can leave you at risk for back pain, constipation (remember, it's all connected!), and a host of other issues.

You can help your body heal by bringing your awareness to how you move throughout the day, your posture, and your breath.

SOME *DOS* AND *DON'TS* FOR YOUR CORE

- **Don't be a contortionist while you feed.** Use props and pillows for support.

- **Sit on your sitz bones.** Sit with your back straight and put your body weight on your sitz bones instead of your tailbone or lower back.

- **Roll out of bed.** Before engaging your abs to get up, roll to your side, sit, and then get up.

- **Bend your knees when lifting.** Think of it as doing a mini squat.

- **Breathe it out.** Notice when you tense up, and breathe it out. Another way to do this is to take audible exhales throughout the day—whenever, wherever. It may feel silly at first, but it is a great way to ensure you are releasing throughout the day! Ahhhh!

Pelvic floor specialists, physical therapists, and/or Pilates instructors that specialize in diastasis recti may all be able to help! (See pg 201)

WHAT IF . . .
I DON'T HAVE ENOUGH MILK?

This is a big one. Breast/chest-feeding horror stories abound—and, OMG, the pressure! But this is another one of those things you can't fully control, so breathe a sigh of relief. While watching videos and reading can be helpful (see pg 248), the truth is that your situation is going to be very unique to your body and baby—here we go again—and most of lactation is really learn-as-you-go. Still, here are some things that are important to keep in mind for maintaining your supply.

Please note, this page is not intended to push you into breast/chest-feeding. As with everything else, *individual decision-making* comes into play! The only "right" choice is the one that's *right for you*. You can breast/chest-feed. You can use formula. You can do both. All is good.

If You Have a Placenta, You Have Milk.

When you hear that someone couldn't breast/chest-feed and there were no birth or postpartum complications or other risk factors (more on this later), typically one or more of the following happened:

1. They didn't or couldn't start feeding soon enough.

2. They didn't or couldn't feed often enough.

3. They didn't have support.

4. They chose not to breast/chest-feed.

Let's break these down.

STARTING EARLY

As soon as you birth the placenta, your body starts producing more prolactin, which in turn means you're making more colostrum. This is true for everyone! But remember, lactation works on a feedback loop (see pg 91)—and that loop needs to be initiated, and continued, by some kind of suck or suction on your nipple. That stimulation is what tells your body to continue making prolactin once the placenta is gone. So, the sooner you can get this conversation going, the better.

This doesn't mean that baby comes out, and BOOM onto the nip they go. There isn't a *huge* rush here—both you and baby just went through something *big*. Give yourself time to adjust, get comfortable, and for the room to not be so busy. Typically babies latch on within the first one to two hours after being born.

But if this doesn't happen for you, don't despair! Not all babies are ready to latch on right away, and you might need some time to catch your breath before you're ready to give it a try. Until you're both ready, hanging out skin to skin and letting baby start sniffing, licking, and sucking at and around the nipple are all very helpful to get things started.

Q: **What if we are separated after birth?**

A: If for whatever reason you are unable to start feeding within the first couple of hours, this does not mean that you can't breast/chest-feed later. But you will want to get the feedback loop started, so it is recommended to either hand express (see pg 248) or to start using a pump. It is possible to collect your colostrum to feed to your baby via a syringe, spoon, or cup so that you don't have to introduce a bottle.

Q: **How do I know if I should hand express or use a pump?**

A: If you are collecting your colostrum to feed to your baby, hand express. Colostrum is thick and can get stuck in the pump. If you are separated from your baby for an extended period of time or not able to bring them to your breast/chest to feed regularly, the pump can be a great way to further stimulate, as hand expressing can get tiring! Once your mature milk comes in, you can stick to the pump if you wish.

Q: **What if I have a C-section?**

A: For some people, surgery has zero impact on their milk. For others, it can mean an extra few days before your mature milk comes down. If your mature milk is delayed and your baby is losing too much weight, supplementation can be a helpful bridge until it comes in. This does not mean you have failed at breast/chest-feeding! It simply means you need to give your body a little more time to get there. You can continue to bring baby to your breast/chest as you supplement, as well as use the pump or hand express to further stimulate as needed.

FEEDING OFTEN

Forget those lactation cookies. The best way to keep up your supply is to feed or pump often. In the beginning, baby needs to be fed every 2–3 hours from the *start* of the last feed, for 15–40 minutes per feed. Yes, that's a whole lot of feeding! But your baby's stomach is tiny when they are first born—about the size of a cherry— and so they need to eat often and in small portions.

Remember, each side of your chest works on its own feedback loop, so you need to give both the same amount of love. We recommend trying to tap both sides in each feed, waiting until the first feels somewhat empty before switching. If this isn't possible, mark where you left off, and be sure to start on the opposite side for the next feed.

#BrilliantTIP

Keep a hair tie or rubber band on your wrist to indicate which side you need to tend to next. There are also apps to keep track.

Q: **That sounds superintense. Is this the rest of my breast/chest-feeding life?**

A: No! As baby gets more efficient, feeding sessions will get shorter and you'll be able to let more time pass in between. When does this happen? It is different for everyone—you probably knew we were gonna say that—but generally if the following things are in place after the first couple of weeks, you can pat yourself on the back and start taking cues from the baby instead of following a set schedule:

- You are not in pain: your nipples and breast/chest overall are not killing you. (If they are, please see a lactation consultant!)
- Baby is continually gaining proper weight.
- Baby is pooping at least three times a day.
- Baby is peeing at least six times a day.

#BrilliantBIT

Sometimes babies cluster feed. This means they show signs of wanting to eat almost nonstop. This is normal newborn behavior! It often happens in the evenings and can be followed by baby sleeping for longer than they normally do. (Baby might want to feed from 7 to midnight and then sleep until 5 a.m.) Some people say it has to do with the growth spurts common around weeks 3, 6, and 9 or simply part of the "witching hour." So long as what's listed above is true for you, it isn't an indication that baby isn't getting enough milk.

LINING UP SUPPORT

Just because breast/chest-feeding is biological, doesn't mean it is easy! Remember to build your squad ahead of time (pg 199). If any of the below apply to you, and you have interest in breast/chest-feeding, we recommend connecting with a lactation consultant prior to labor as these are the instances where supply is most often affected:

- Insufficient glandular tissue (hypoplastic breasts)
- Polycystic ovary syndrome (PCOS)
- Hypothyroidism
- A previous breast/chest surgery
- Prior radiation treatment for breast/chest cancer

A NOTE ON VERY FLAT OR INVERTED NIPPLES

While this doesn't affect production, if you have very flat or inverted nipples (meaning, the actual nipple doesn't extend from the areola), baby may need some extra help finding a latch. It is possible that post-birth, your nipples will end up coming out more than you are used to, but we still recommend you connect with a consultant ahead of time just in case, as they may be able to help you prepare.

169

A NOTE ON THE BODY-MIND CONNECTION

If you experience postpartum depression, anxiety, or extreme stress, your milk supply can be affected. Be sure to reach out to a therapist specializing in the perinatal period in addition to an IBCLC (International Board Certified Lactation Consultant) if breast/chest-feeding is something you wish to maintain. If breast/chest-feeding is what is causing your anxiety, it's okay to decide that it is not the right choice for you! Nothing is better than your baby getting to actually experience *you*.

Want more information? Check out our top tips for breast/chest-feeding on pg 228!

Supplementation and Formula-Feeding

There are some things to know if you're using formula or donated milk to supplement breast/chest-feeding or to exclusively feed your babe:

- **How often?** As with breast/chest-feeding, you want to follow baby's lead, look out for hunger cues (see pg 173), and be flexible with the schedule. If baby looks hungry, *feed* them. Otherwise, generally you want to feed your newborn every two to three hours.

- **How much?** Newborns need very little formula when they are first born—about half an ounce per feeding for the first couple days. By the end of the first week they'll need 1–2 ounces per bottle. After two or three weeks, they'll eat about 2–3 ounces each time.[114] After the first month they might need four ounces. On average, your baby should take in about 2½ ounces (75 mL) of formula a day for every pound (453 g) of body weight.[115] See pg 249 for more resources on bottle-feeding.

- **How to give the bottle?** Letting your baby lead—again!—is important here. You want the baby to be able to regulate how much milk they get, just as they do when they breast/chest-feed. To a certain extent, you want to try to mimic what they would do at the breast, so instead of *giving them* the bottle you should let them *take the bottle*. Feed them upright and hold the bottle horizontally (just tip it slightly) instead of vertically, so baby can control the flow. They will take breaks and push the nipple away from time to time. Check out pg 248 for more info on *Paced Bottle-Feeding*.

○ **Which formula?** For the most part, it doesn't matter which brand you choose. They are all very similar. Just make sure it's made for infants, i.e. under one year, and learn how to safely prep a bottle. (See pg 248 for resources on this.) If you notice baby is having digestive issues, talk to your pediatrician about trying a different brand.

WHAT IF . . .
I IRREVERSIBLY MESS UP MY BABY?

You've spent *all this time* focusing on your pregnancy and planning for your birth . . . and then it hits you: *I need to take care of this baby . . . forever?!*

We know that this can feel like *a lot. But you don't need to know everything at once.*

It's *impossible* to know everything at once because you first need to meet your babe—which you can't do until they arrive (duh). And then, once you do, they are going to be changing *all the time*. Just when you think you've nailed something down, it will change again. Remember, it's not about the path, it's how we move through it.

Here are some tools to help you gain confidence and have a starting place to build from.

Basic Safety

ARE THEY GETTING ENOUGH MILK?

Here's a very simplified guide to know that your baby is getting enough.

#BrilliantBIT

If you are breast/chest-feeding, babies can't overfeed themselves! They will only eat as much as they need.

WEIGHT: While it is normal for baby to lose up to 7–10 percent of their weight in the first few days, by the end of the fourteenth day or so they should be back at their birth weight and gaining approximately ⅔ to 1⅓ ounces daily from there, depending on their body weight.

POOPS: On day one there should be at least one poop, and on day 2, two poops. By day 3 or 4, and moving forward, there should be at least three-plus poops in a twenty-four-hour period. There may be twelve—and that's okay!—but generally you don't want it to dip below three. If it does, it can be a sign of dehydration.

PEES: This can be hard to discern sometimes if mixed in with the poop, but it follows a similar pattern. By day 4 though, you should see six-plus wet diapers per day.

If all these things are happening for you, breathe easy. If not, it's a good idea to check in with your pediatrician. This is not a poor reflection on you. In fact, your paying attention is a sign of really, really good parenting.

#BrilliantBIT

A note on poop color—baby's poop will turn from brown (meconium) to greenish/yellowish to yellow (and seedy in consistency) once your mature milk is in. You may also notice as time goes on that the poop becomes green again. This isn't a huge deal, sometimes it just happens, but if you are concerned or notice mucus or blood in the poo, let your pediatrician know.

HUNGER CUES

Remember, your baby is here to help you learn them! Learning to read their hunger cues will help you feed them before a full-on meltdown happens. Here's generally how it goes:

I'm Hungry.

- Starts licking and making smacking sounds—aka opening and closing mouth
- Sucks on hands, clothes, toys—anything nearby really
- Starts rooting—aka moving head side to side or front to back (it looks kind of freaky if you don't know what it is at first)

Feed Me Now.

- Fist to mouth
- Gets squirmy or fidgety
- Breathing is faster
- Positions themselves near the breast/chest

Meltdown!—Too Hungry to Eat, Love Me First.

- Fussing
- Agitated movements
- Frantic
- Full-on crying and freaking out!

Notice that crying is usually the *last* sign of wanting to eat. So see if you can catch them before the meltdown begins!

IS MY BABY TOO HOT OR TOO COLD?

The general rule of thumb is to put baby in one more layer than would be comfortable for you. So if you are wearing a t-shirt, they should have a onesie and a shirt. The best way to check if you baby is too hot or cold? Touch the back of their neck to see if it is sweaty and their hands and feet to see if they are too cold. A lot of people go crazy making sure their house is exactly the right temperature, the humidifier is perfect, etc. There's no need to go that far. If you're worried, the best way to help your baby regulate their temperature is to hold them skin to skin.

IS MY BABY STILL BREATHING?

You'll probably check a thousand times. Especially for those who have experienced loss, this may feel impossible to let go of. There's probably nothing we can say here to prevent you from doing this, but do know that because your baby's lungs are brand-new, it may look like they are struggling to breathe—their chest may move up and down dramatically, they make some wacky sounds—but this is just their lungs learning how to work!

WHERE AND HOW SHOULD MY BABY SLEEP?

The safest way for babies to sleep is on their back—not on their stomach or side—on a firm surface, without secondhand smoke of any kind, and with no blankets, pillows, or stuffed animals around. The American Academy of Pediatrics also recommends room sharing for the first six months of the baby's life.

That being said, a lot of people end up sharing their bed with their newborns, either sometimes or all the time, since it can allow you both to rest more throughout the night. If this is you, just make sure you are doing it safely! Co-sleeping is not safe on a couch or anyplace other than a bed with a firm mattress. It's also not recommended if you are not breast/chest-feeding, if you or your partner smoke, or if either of you have taken anything that can make you drowsy. There should be no pillows, crevices, or blankets near baby's face. See pg 174 for more info on safely bed-sharing with a newborn.

WAKE UP YOUR BABY!

It is not normal or expected for a newborn to sleep through the night. For the first few weeks the priority is establishing a healthy weight and feeding pattern, so do not let your baby sleep more than a few hours at a time. If they are sleeping more than three hours, it may actually be an indication that they are not getting enough milk. Wake them up! Once you know your baby is gaining the proper weight, producing enough diapers, and is not jaundiced or dehydrated, then it is okay to stretch it a bit to give yourself more of a break if baby will let you. But remember, if you're breast/chest-feeding, you are still on that feedback loop, so even if your baby wants to sleep for longer stretches, you breasts/chest might need emptying.

PSA: YOU CAN'T SPOIL A NEWBORN.

Your newborn is biologically incapable of self-soothing, which makes you—and the humans around you—pretty much your babe's sole comfort measure. You are not creating "bad habits" by responding to their cries or even holding them 24/7. You are actually teaching them that they are safe! In fact, research tells us there are lots of benefits of early skin-to-skin contact between parents and babies, especially if they are born premature,[116] including better breast/chest-feeding outcomes,[117] less crying, and stabler heart rates, breathing, and blood sugar levels.[118,119] Get snuggling!

Once your baby starts exhibiting signs of self-soothing, then it is appropriate to allow them to start soothing themselves. This looks different for everyone, so let your baby lead and keep checking your Gut as to how to best respond. You'll know!

WHAT IF . . .
I NEVER SLEEP AGAIN?

No beating around the bush on this one—your sleep pattern is about to be rocked. But you can do this! Your body *does* adapt, eventually your kid *will* sleep, and we're about to give you some tips to help you survive.

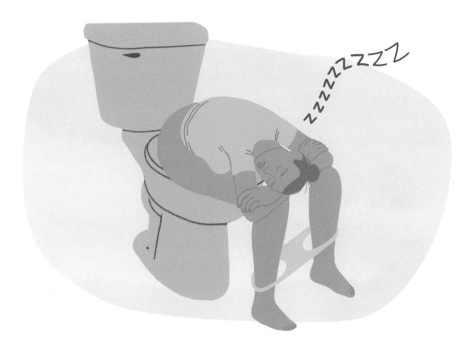

Surviving Sleep Deprivation

RECALIBRATE YOUR SLEEP SCHEDULE.

Newborns need about sixteen hours of sleep every day, including nighttime sleep.[120] This means that you have sixteen hours of opportunity! But because newborn's circadian rhythms are not yet established, they may sleep for most of the day and wake during the night (womp womp). It can be hard to adjust your rhythm to this, but the biggest tip for survival here is to *sleep when your baby sleeps!* These daytime siestas will be your saviors and are key to getting you through those first weeks. For you naysayers: *I have SO many other things to do . . . I can't nap . . .* You can! We promise. Here are some ways to make it happen.

- Prioritize naps over chores or screen time. You really, really can get that other stuff done another time—or ask someone to do it for you! Actually, if you let yourself rest, you can probably get the other stuff done more efficiently later on.

- Keep time with visitors short so you can rest. Or if you feel ready, ask them to stay a bit and watch baby while *you* sleep.

- If you have a partner or helper, take turns "sleeping in." One takes the baby to the other room while the other gets some z's.

- Have some soothing music, meditations, playlists, white noise, etc., ready to go to help you drift off.

- Rest as you feed. Even if you aren't sleeping, allow yourself to relax instead of scrolling through your phone. If you're breast/chest-feeding, try doing some feeds while you are lying down (remember safe co-sleeping recommendations) so you can kill two birds with one stone.

#BrilliantTIP

You don't *have* to change all those diapers at night! It's totally fine to skip a change to let yourself sleep a little bit more. We're not saying let them swim in their poo for hours, but they've been in water for the last ten months . . . they'll be okay for a tiny bit longer. (Just watch out for diaper rash.)

Helping Baby Sleep

In addition to ensuring *you* get some daytime z's, here's how you can support your baby in getting some z's of their own.

LET YOUR BABY LEAD YOU.

As you get to know your baby, you'll start to see when they are hungry vs. when they are sleepy vs. when they have gas. It might take time, but you'll get there—even if at first it all seems like a puzzle.

Learning to understand when your babe is getting sleepy will help you help them fall asleep before they start howling. Some signs that can indicate your baby is ready to sleep include:

- Pulling their ears
- Blank stares
- Yawning
- Rubbing their eyes
- Hiccups
- Jerky movements

SLEEP BRINGS MORE SLEEP.

Letting your baby stay up for longer during the day does not mean they will sleep more at night. In general it is best to not let newborns be up for more than 2–3 hours at a time. Our bodies produce cortisol when we are awake and too much of this hormone can cause hyperactivity, hyperstimulation, and inhibit the release of melatonin, which can make going to sleep harder for little babies—and adults![121] When we nap, our levels of cortisol are reduced, and we get a reset that makes it easier to fall asleep again. So the more often your baby naps, the better they will nap again! The soothing tips on pg 177 may also help put your babe to bed.

HOLD THEM.

Babies *love* falling asleep in your arms or right next to you, and they will often sleep for longer if they are held. This is normal behavior—it doesn't mean you are spoiling your baby. You're just making sleep easier for everyone involved! If this doesn't work for you, try using a swaddle. This can help the baby feel safe and cozy and more ready to snooze while not being held.

#BrilliantTIP

A note on swaddling—while some babies love to feel snug as a bug in a rug, others may not dig the swaddle so much. If your baby is not into it, try leaving their arms free so they have access to their hands and more freedom to move.

SLEEP TRAINING

We totally understand the desire to get your baby sleeping ASAP. There are so many philosophies and theories about sleep training—we aren't here to debate them. At this stage, we just want to point out what we feel is important for you to keep in mind as you do your research:

- Every baby is different—just in case you haven't heard this one from us enough. So not all babies need "sleep training" because some might be sleeping just fine without it.
- There is no "right time" to start.
- Not all babies *can* be sleep trained—even if you follow all the recommendations down to a tee. And it's okay if sleep training isn't right for your family.
- It is not recommended to start sleep training in the first few weeks. (Remember, babies don't have any self-soothing techniques yet!)

There are hundreds of books and programs out there on sleep. Don't let them stress you out. Focus on following your baby's rhythms and trust your Gut for what your family needs. Individual decision-making, baby!

179

WHAT IF . . .
MY BABY NEVER STOPS CRYING?

We know it can be heartbreaking to watch those little lips quiver and feel like you can't or don't know how to help them. It's so hard!

An important thing to know is that when baby cries, it doesn't always mean something is wrong, they need their diaper changed, or they are hungry or in pain. Crying is a normal psychological phase babies move through, and sometimes they just need to be comforted. This is a whole new world for them, so they need to be assured, and reassured, and reassured again that this place is safe for them and they have support when they get stuck. (*Hey, does that sound familiar?!*)

Eventually you may learn to read your babies' different cries and cues, quickly discerning what they mean, but in the meantime doing what you can to mimic the feeling of being in a womb is helpful for them.

Here are some soothing methods you can rely on to cycle through.

- Being skin to skin
- Exaggerated and repetitive movements like rocking, bouncing, or swaying—bouncing on the birth ball with the babe can work wonders!
- White noise—use an app, get a white noise machine, shush, or bring the babe near running water in a pinch.
- Sucking—on your breast/chest, a pacifier, your fingers, or their hands. Anything, works really!

A NOTE ON COLIC, OR EXCESSIVE CRYING

Normal infants cry anywhere from one to two hours per day in the first six weeks of life.[122] If your baby is inconsolable or crying excessively, check in with your pediatrician to ensure that nothing is going on physically.

Colic is when your baby cries excessively and persistently and there's no clear reason why. The medical community disagrees on what causes colic: *Is there actually physical discomfort? Are all babies "colicy" but some just need more help "turning off" their cry?* Because definitions are different, it is hard to gauge exactly how many babies cry more often than is expected. Call it colic, call it *Help! I can't get my baby to stop crying* . . . It can take an emotional toll on the family. If this is you, get support. While colic typically clears on its own by age 3–4 months, that's a lot of crying to suffer through! Remember, taking care of yourself *is* taking care of your baby.

WHAT IF . . .
I GET POSTPARTUM DEPRESSION?

Here's the cosmic joke about having a baby: You have just grown and carried around another human being for almost ten months. All your organs and hormones shifted to accommodate this. Then you have to do the most physically challenging thing you'll likely ever do to get that baby out. *Then* you have to take care of said baby *with your body* at the same time you are healing that same body from the aforementioned ten months of pregnancy, *plus* whatever happened during the birth . . . while you have the brand-new responsibility of keeping a teeny, tiny, seemingly defenseless baby alive, on very little sleep, while potentially facing some serious identity shifts—with your hormones going haywire all the while.

Yes, there *are* going to be some emotional ups and down for the first bunch of weeks post-birth!

> ### #BrilliantBIT
> One of the biggest hormonal shifts happens the day your mature milk comes in. Cue the uncontrollable tears. This tends to fall around day 3–5 postpartum, and for those giving birth in a hospital, it often coincides with the day you get discharged. So heads up, it can be a rough day! Cry it out.

We encourage you to let yourself feel all the feels—and that might include feeling downright nuts at times. This is normal, but that doesn't mean it is easy. The postpartum period can feel lonely, like all the responsibility falls on you and you can't escape. For some people, these feelings—and hormones—can start to interfere with your day-to-day and your ability to care for yourself or others.

Postpartum depression affects approximately one in nine birthing people[123]—though it's likely an even higher number since many cases go undiagnosed. While there are some people at increased risk (see below), anyone can experience it . . . including partners!

PPD is not a reflection of you as a parent or person—just a sign that you could use some support.

WHAT ARE SOME SIGNS TO LOOK OUT FOR?

- Feeling sad or depressed most of the time
- Inability to focus on simple tasks
- Insomnia or nightmares that keep you up
- Compulsive eating or lack of appetite
- Extreme or consistent ups and downs after sixish weeks

- Feelings of hopelessness or an extreme lack of motivation
- Feelings of wanting to harm yourself or your baby
- Avoidance of baby
- Racing obsessive scary or negative thoughts
- Fear of leaving the house or being alone with the baby

- Suicidal thoughts
- Disorientation and confusion
- Obsessive thoughts about your baby
- Hallucinations
- Paranoia
- Attempts to harm yourself or baby

Very important note: There are a whole host of perinatal mood and anxiety disorders (PMAD)—some more severe than others. Even if you are just feeling a *little* anxious, or depressed, or unsure, it is still worth it to seek support! The Edinburgh Postpartum Depression scale is a useful self-assessment tool (see pg 248), most effective if done periodically so you can see if you are improving or worsening over time. Most people don't realize that the onset for symptoms can be up to two years.

Getting By

Simply normalizing that the postpartum period is not all warm fuzzies can be freeing in and of itself. But postpartum depression or not, this period can just be effing hard. Here are some things to help you out.

PLAN AHEAD.

While anyone can experience postpartum depression, there are a few indicators that you may be at a higher risk:

- History of anxiety or depression, or other mental health conditions
- You've had PPD before.
- Traumatic birth
- Stressful events over the last year
- Your baby has special needs.
- Financial struggles
- Lack of support or problems with your partner
- Difficulty feeding
- Unplanned or unwanted pregnancy

Get your squad ready! (See pg 199.)

AVOID CABIN FEVER.

You will likely be in your home for many more hours than you are used to. Have distractions around. Movies, podcasts, audiobooks, TV shows . . . For some, keeping craft projects or puzzles around can be fun—though don't put pressure on yourself to get much done. These diversions are meant to allow you to briefly breathe and reconnect with yourself. Also, reread page 158 for tips on your shifting identity.

GET MOVING!

We know finding the time to exercise may seem impossible—or the last thing you want to do!—but it can save you. In fact, exercise has been proven to be as effective as antidepressants in treating postpartum depression.[124] One, two, three, break!

MEDICATION

In some cases, and with the support of your therapist and care provider, antidepressants can help. There are meds that are safe to use while breast/chest-feeding, just be sure to ask your practitioner. And if you go on antidepressants during this period, it doesn't mean you'll need them forever.

Repeat after Us . . .

IT'S TEMPORARY AND LEGIT.

Keep reminding yourself that what you are feeling is temporary and that there are real legitimate reasons for your feelings. Though while you are *in it,* it can feel like forever, the craziness *will* change. This *won't* be forever.

YOU'RE GOING TO FUCK UP.

The transition to parenthood doesn't happen overnight—or even in a few weeks. You are constantly going to be learning. You *are* going to fuck up, so don't bother striving for perfection. Instead, strive for patience, kindness, awareness, and growth.

WHAT IF . . .
I NEVER WANT TO HAVE SEX AGAIN?

It's totally okay if . . .

- You really don't feel like having sex.
- You have trouble reaching orgasm.
- Your breasts/chest leak during sex.
- You have trouble getting wet.
- The thought of your baby needing you distracts you during sex.
- You'd rather sleep.
- Having the baby in the same room while you have sex freaks you out.
- You don't feel sexy.

Here are some reasons you may experience a change in your sex drive—though it doesn't mean it's dead, we promise!

HORMONES

Hormone shifts play a major role in how you feel sexually postpartum, particularly if you are breast/chest-feeding since that prolactin can affect your estrogen and progesterone production, which can result in a lower libido.[125] Add these hormonal changes to the stress of being a new parent and zap—there goes your sex drive. In some ways this shift is designed by nature: you're wired to care for your baby as opposed to making a new one.

IT JUST DOESN'T FEEL GOOD.

Lower levels of estrogen can cause vaginal dryness, making sex less comfortable. While this generally gets resolved with time, lube definitely helps in the meantime (and always, really).

It is also possible, especially if there was trauma during your birth, that your *fear* of insertion or any vaginal play (*Will my perineaum tear again? It looks like a wreck down there. . . . What about my hemorrhoids?*) is the root cause of physical symptoms like vaginal tightness, making penetration of any kind painful or impossible. If any of this resonates or if you are feeling any pain during sex, go see a pelvic floor specialist. Sex *can* feel good again! And that pain may be an indication that your body needs some help healing.

BREAST/CHEST-FEEDING

In addition to the hormonal shifts it brings, breast/chest-feeding can also change your relationship to your body—you may feel touched-out, the fact that you can lactate may make you feel disconnected from your body, and/or it may feel strange or wrong to include your breasts/chest as part of your sexuality when your baby needs them. There is no magic solution here, but simply recognizing where you are and communicating this with your partner are a good first step.

#BrilliantTIP

If you are having trouble including your breasts/chest in your sexuality, try giving them different identities for their different roles. Maybe you call them one thing while feeding and another during sex. Maybe you use your milk as a part of role-playing, instead of quickly getting rid of it or ignoring it. The main thing to get across here is that it is not dirty or shameful for both your baby and your partner to derive pleasure from the same part of you. And drawing the distinction when they are playing each role can be helpful.

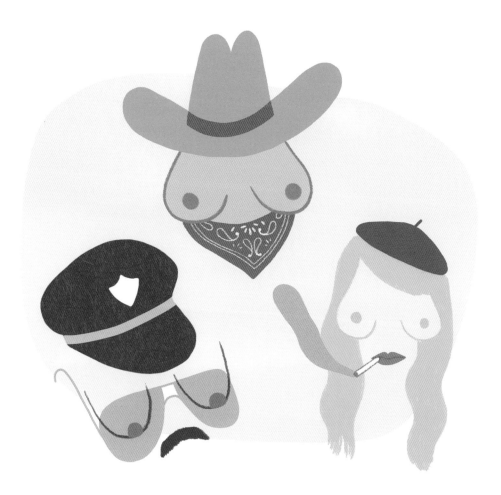

YOUR EMOTIONAL STATE

If you're experiencing postpartum depression, anxiety, PTSD, or just having an overall hard time, it is very common for your sex life to be affected. Communicate with your partner and give yourself some time to heal. There's also just plain ole *exhaustion*. This can have a big impact too. Get support as needed, and remember, you won't be stuck here forever.

Getting Your Groove Back

While your body may feel different, different doesn't have to be detrimental. Just as there may be things that don't feel so good anymore, there are likely many new pleasures for you to discover and explore! Here are some tips to help you get your groove back.

- **Masturbate.** This is a great way to get comfortable with your post-birth body and start to safely explore what you do and do not like. Challenge yourself to even have some fun with this—after all, you have a new body to explore. What can you find?! Share your discoveries with your partner if you feel comfortable.

- **Communicate.** Let your partner know as soon as something doesn't feel good. And let them know when you do like something. If you have found something on your own that you like, ask for it.

- **Experiment.** Now that you have this different-feeling body, you might as well take it for a joyride! Get some new toys. Use lube. Try role-playing. Live out a new fantasy. Allow yourself to go a little wild in your new identity.

- **Just get back on the horse.** And we say this with care. This doesn't mean neglecting your feelings or that they don't matter. We know you are exhausted. But sometimes it takes *being intimate* to remember that you actually really like it.

WHAT IF . . .
I DON'T FEEL READY TO GO BACK TO WORK?

The reality of—our lack of—parental leave in the United States is grim, to say the least. We're the only industrialized country with no national family leave policy. And this means that one in four birthing parents have to go back to work only ten days (ten!) after childbirth.[126] And while the Family and Medical Leave Act of 1993[127] requires twelve weeks of leave for *qualifying* employees—think full-time workers of *big* companies only—it's still often *unpaid*. And so, even if you're one of the "lucky" ones entitled to those twelve weeks, you might not be able to afford to take the time off anyway. And what happens if you work part-time or as a freelancer with no benefits? The financial stress of having a child is huge regardless of the type of work you do. That's not to mention the lack of affordable child care options most new parents are faced with.

This is all true in the United States, despite the data and research confirming that paid parental leave not only reduces infant mortality and improves health outcomes, but that it is possible to support working families without harming businesses.[128] And yet, most working parents are faced with the choice of returning to work too soon, leaving the workforce for some time or forever, or having huge financial expenses to pay for child care.

This all sucks.

While nothing we say will make the transition back to work that much easier or help you decide when or if to go back at all, we still want to address this big what-if and loudly say: *We. Feel. You.*

Here are some things to think about:

FEEDING BABY

- ○ If you're breast/chest-feeding and going back to work:
  - Practice with the bottle for at least two weeks before you need to go back. Some babies are finicky and prefer one bottle to another or one nipple to another, so get that experimenting in first. Some babies won't take the bottle at all at first. Give yourself plenty of time to practice so that you don't have to feel as stressed when you actually do need to go.
  - Start building your breast/chest milk reserves about 2–3 weeks before going back to work. See pg 230 for pumping tips.
  - Make sure your work has a place to pump and a place for you to store your milk. Learn your rights as a breast/chest-feeding employee. (See pg 230.)
- ○ If you're bottle-feeding make sure whoever is taking care of your baby knows how to feed them: how often, how much, etc. . . . see pg 230 for more.

CHILD CARE

While we can't tell you if hiring a nanny, doing a nanny-share, sending your babe to day care, or leaving them with friends/family is the right choice for you, what we can say is babies thrive from being around other babies and other adults. And so, even if it seems hard to imagine being separated from them or having someone else take care of them, know that it is likely going to feel harder for you than it actually is for them. (Sorry!)

OH, THE GUILT!

Our midwife friend says you give birth to a baby—and guilt. No matter what you decide to do, you'll probably feel you're not doing enough: not spending enough time at work, not spending enough time with your baby, not spending enough time with your partner, family, and friends, not spending enough time at the gym, and on and on and on. All we can say is: *Holy crap, you're doing so much already.* Work on setting boundaries so you don't feel as stretched (e.g., skip the office party or the playdate on the weekend). *You don't have to do it all. The best gift you can give yourself is the credit that you're doing your best.* Even when—especially when—you feel like you're not.

PUMP LOUD AND PROUD.

We know it can be really hard to pump at work. Maybe you're quarantined to a closet. Maybe you know others can hear you. Maybe you're the first employee to have a kid so everyone else just doesn't get it. And maybe you can feel all those eyes on you—rolling or staring you down because you have *"the luxury"* of pumping while they have to answer emails. We must model the respect we deserve to get. We know this isn't easy, but the more of us that can pump loud and proud, the more normalized it will become. And then we'll see who is rolling their eyes at whom.

part

5

YOUR TOOLS
TO RETURN TO

WHILE WE HOPE YOU OF COURSE READ THIS BOOK COVER TO COVER, we wanted to put all of our top tips, tools, and suggestions in one place for you to easily return to as needed.

This is also a good place for your support peeps to visit so that they too can arm themselves to help you along the way.

CAN YOUR BIRTH PLACE AND CARE PROVIDERS ACTUALLY GIVE YOU WHAT YOU NEED?

While you certainly have rights as a pregnant person (see pg 51), it's still vital to consider what your *viable choices actually are* where and with whom you've chosen to give birth. And though you can refuse any treatment (you own your body after all!), if you are birthing in a hospital, there are institutional policies in place that can make it harder for you to do so without consequences. Plus, the power dynamics at play in the birth room can be strong—it's hard to speak up for yourself and exercise your rights to informed consent (see pg 50) when you are naked and in labor! So make sure you and your clinical care and birth place are truly aligned in advance. Here are some questions to help you figure it out:

Questions to Make Sure Your Hospital Can Best Support You

- Can my partner stay overnight postpartum?
- How many support people can be in the labor room with me?
- What is your policy for eating and drinking during labor?

o Can my support people stay with me if I get an epidural or need to go to the OR?

o Do you have birth balls and peanut balls or do I need to bring my own?

o Are there any protocols that would require separation between me and the baby?

o If I decide to keep my placenta, can I take it home with me? What are the hospital protocols regarding this?

o Does your staff have any special LGBTQ+ training?

o Do you have baths and/or showers in the labor rooms that I can use while in labor?

o Do you offer breast/chest-feeding classes immediately postpartum?

o Do you have lactation consultants on staff? How often are they there?

o As long as everyone is healthy, can my baby stay with me at all times postpartum?

o What level NICU do you have in your hospital? What happens if my baby needs more attention than your unit can provide?

Deciding Between a Midwife and an OBGYN

There is a ton of misunderstanding around what midwives actually do. Midwives are clinical providers that support birth in hospital settings, birth centers, and at home. That's right, you can work with a midwife in a hospital! And, many midwifery-led births employ the use of pain medication, as per patient preference.

Midwives are trained to view health care as a collaborative process. While obstetric education involves learning a myriad of skills to *manage complications* of birth, typically in a one-size-fits-most model, midwifery education is all about viewing birth as a normal event. They are there to facilitate the process and

195

provide individualized care informed by a person's social and psychological history to the same degree as their medical history. They are also trained to identify medical and obstetric complications and consult and refer to obstetricians as indicated. If a serious complication does arise unexpectedly, midwives can comanage your care with an obstetrician to ensure medical needs are met. Thanks, OBs!

Working with a midwife also lessens your chance of having an episiotomy, vacuum/forceps delivery, and C-section while increasing the likelihood of being satisfied with your birth.[129] So, while there are certainly some fabulous OBGYNs out there, if you are low-risk, look into your midwifery options too! But even with midwives, you still need to use the guide below to ensure they are the best support for you.

Questions to Ask Your Care Provider When You're Birthing in a Hospital

- Will you be at my labor? At what point of labor do you show up? Do you stay with me until baby is born? *This is especially important if you're working with a big practice.*

- What is your C-section rate and what factors do you think contribute to it?

- Do you support VBACs (vaginal birth after C-section)? *Even if you are having your first child, the answer to this will give you a sense of how conservative the practice is.*

- How do you feel about a doula joining my birth team? *Again, even if you don't plan on having one, the answer will give you a feel for the provider.*

- If my water breaks before contractions begin, what is your protocol from there? How long until I need to come to the hospital? (See pg 109 for more info on this one.)

- How long past my due date can I go before being induced?
- Can I be intermittently monitored instead of continuously monitored, for the entirety of my labor, if I have no interventions and everyone is looking healthy? (See pg 144.)
- Can I use the shower or bath in the hospital labor room?
- Am I limited in my pushing positions at any time during the pushing phase?
- If both the baby and I are healthy, do you have a limit on how long I can push for?
- Do you support delayed cord clamping? (See pg 73 for resources on this.)
- Do you support "gentle cesareans" or "family-centered cesareans"? (See pg 145.)
- What does your postpartum care look like—immediately and in the days/weeks that follow birth?

For those who are hoping to have an unmedicated birth and are choosing to go to a hospital, the following are superimportant:

- Having a heplock instead of IV so you have more freedom to move around
- Being intermittently monitored instead of continuously monitored
- Being able to use the shower or bath in the labor room
- Being able to eat and drink throughout
- They won't push an induction on you before 42 weeks.
- They are open to working with a doula.
- They aren't asking you to come to the hospital as soon as your water breaks so long as you are GBS negative, the fluids are clear, and no other health factors are at play.

Questions to Ask Home Birth
or Birth Center Midwives

- What is your training and licensing?

- At what point do you come to my home? And who comes with you? (For home births)

- What is your transfer rate? What typically accounts for most of your transfers?

- In uncertain situations, do you tend to lean more toward transferring or staying home? Why?

- What happens if my baby is breech?

- How far past my due date can I go before needing to get induced? How does transfer of care happen if this is the case?

- What disqualifies me from your care? What happens then?

- Do you have a relationship with any hospitals in the area in case a transfer is necessary?

- Do you stay with me if a transfer becomes necessary? What is the protocol if the transfer occurs in labor versus postpartum? What about if the transfer is for baby once born?

- What does your postpartum care look like—immediately and in the days/weeks that follow birth?

- Who handles my postpartum care if a transfer is needed?

BUILDING YOUR DREAM TEAM

Of all times, *this is when to take care of yourself.* And we want to encourage you to shift your mindset when it comes to building your dream team. Think of them more as necessities than accessories. You're not splurging or being spoiled by taking care of yourself; these are the people that can really help you make it through. Use them!

A note on finding a practitioner: It is very important that you find someone specializing in the perinatal period across modalities. Remember your Body and Emotions are different in pregnancy, so you want someone who really gets it—and knows what they are doing! Some insurance companies or flexi spending accounts will cover some or all of the costs, so be sure to check your plan if you have one.

#BrilliantTIP

While all the baby clothes are cute, do you really need another onesie? Consider adding gift certificates for practitioners and services like those described below to your baby gift registry if you have one. Or start one! These resources are truly the best gifts anyone can give you.

Throughout Pregnancy, Birth, and Postpartum

OVERALL SUPPORT

- **Doula,** duh (see page 3 for specifics on what a doula does)!
- **Family members or friends**
  - Who will you feel comfortable hanging out with in the days leading up to your EDD that can help keep you distracted?
  - Who can set up a meal train for you?
  - Who can you rely on and trust to come over on short notice for a real SOS?

- **Partner** and/or other dedicated birth support person

- **Le Leche League and other support groups.** Google around your area. There are IRL groups as well as digital. Often these groups are free or very low cost and a great way to normalize your experience and learn from other parents.

BODY SQUAD

- **Lactation consultant.** If you have reasons to be concerned about your supply or ability to lactate (see pg 165), it may be nice to connect with someone prior to your birth. If you don't fall into this category, we still recommend you keep some names on hand so that you don't need to scramble once your babe is here. There are both lactation counselors and IBCLCs. While counselors can certainly be helpful, IBCLCs have the most training and are the only ones able to diagnose things like tongue-tie. So when possible, we recommend working with an IBCLC.

- **Acupuncturist.** They can ease many ailments you may experience throughout your pregnancy including aches and pains, insomnia, stress, and nausea. Some can also prepare herbal blends for continued support and uterine toning. They can be especially useful to see in the weeks leading up to your EDD to help your body prep for labor and, in some cases, get the party started. When you are ready postpartum, they are also around to help you heal.

- **Webster technique–based chiropractor.** You know all that talk about baby's position in regards to labor progression? Well these guys are some of your best defense to help address your pelvic alignment. They can help create more space for baby to position themselves most optimally. A chiropractor can assist with any hip or pelvic imbalances to create more space for baby to come down and help your Body feel less icky during pregnancy. They will also help you feel better in your body postpartum.

- **Massage therapist.** Need we say more? While a massage can certainly feel like a treat, it's actually a really productive way to support your body coping through pregnancy and preparing for labor. Plus, it just feels so damn good. Give this to yourself postpartum too—with all that feeding and carrying you will be sore!

- **Pelvic floor specialist.** In many countries, pelvic floor rehabilitation is part of postpartum care, but not in the United States. Your pelvic floor is not only responsible for the health of your vaginal muscles, but remember, it also helps guard against incontinence, painful intercourse, constipation, and any organ prolapse later on. That's kind of a big deal! A specialist will help you understand where your unique pelvic floor is and give you personalized exercises to strengthen or loosen your hammock. We recommend having a session at least once in pregnancy before labor and then again postpartum.

- **Herbalist and/or holistic nutritionist or health coach.** Ensuring you are eating whole, nutrient-rich foods and good fats is vital to tissue health as well as a healthy pregnancy and to help prevent against some postpartum discomforts like constipation. Herbs can be a great addition to further support your Body as it is working overtime in pregnancy and then healing from all the hormonal shifts and physical changes postpartum.

EMOTIONAL SUPPORT

- **Mental health professional.** Did you know that during your first trimester, you are getting about 400 birth control pills worth of progesterone a day?![130] Add all these hormonal changes to the big transitions happening overall and things can get . . . *hairy*. Even if you don't experience anxiety or depression, we still recommend that everyone tries to get some emotional support during this time. Try to find a practitioner that has a somatic (Body) element to their practice. Remember you can't always process everything through your Head!

Postpartum-Specific Help

OVERALL SUPPORT

- **Postpartum doula.** Postpartum doulas come to your home and help with your transition to parenthood. Everyone works a little differently, but postpartum doulas can assist with light housework, feeding baby, feeding you, lactation support, pet care, chores, etc. Some postpartum doulas will also do overnight care, helping you with your baby so you can catch some extra z's.

- **Food delivery service or Seamless.** Sometimes you just can't cook or have no food in the freezer to defrost. Give yourself the break.

FOR YOUR PHYSICAL SPACE

A clean and organized living space can actually make you feel more grounded. Even if you are only able to do it once, it's worth it!

- Housecleaning service

- Laundry pickup—if you don't have in your home

- Dog walker (or friend/neighbor)

FOR YOUR BABY

- **Pediatrician.** When possible, we always recommend finding one that has a lactation consultant on staff. Pediatricians are not traditionally trained in lactation. So any questions about feeding should be directed to the IBCLC.

- **Craniosacral therapy.** CST is very gentle touch-based therapy that can help baby with tension or extra pressure from any birth trauma. It can also help with their latching on if their jaw is very tight or they can't turn their head fully in one direction.

RETHINKING STAGES OF LABOR

You've likely read about the "stages of labor" before based on the dilation of your cervix. We'd like to present them to you in a different light; after all, the numbers don't give us that much information anyway (see pg 119) and you can't do cervical exams on your own.

Instead, we want to turn your focus to the *experience* of labor—the key indicators of how the Body and Emotions may change throughout the process—so you can get a sense of where you are without focusing as much on the time or whether you're moving fast enough.

Refer to the Coping Cheat Sheet (see pg 212) to see which coping techniques may prove most useful along the way.

Also keep in mind this is based on physiological birth. Things may feel different if and when interventions are introduced, though you may still be able to note some of these markers. Remember every body is different, so it may not happen exactly like this for you.

GETTING PREPPED:
Is it labor now? Is it labor now? (aka Pre-Labor)

How long: A few weeks to a few days before the onset of labor. Or you may never experience it at all.

Physical Experience

- Increased Braxton-Hicks or "practice contractions"
- Lightning-like sensation in your crotch
- Feeling that baby is "dropping" as baby moves down into pelvis
- Increased vaginal secretions, including losing your mucus plug
- Soft, loose stools, even diarrhea
- Backache, cramping, nausea

Emotional Experience

- Nesting instincts pick up.

- Highs and lows

- Is this it? Is it labor? Is this it? Is this labor?

#BrilliantBIT

Braxton-Hicks or "practice contractions" feel different from labor contractions. B.H. contractions feel like a tightening and release: your belly becomes as hard as a rock, and then it is soft again. Labor contractions have a wave-like shape: building, peaking, and coming down. They will also become longer, stronger, and more consistent over time. Sometimes increased B.H. contractions can be a sign of dehydration, so drink up. While not everyone experiences B.H. contractions, if you do, it's a great opportunity to practice taking nice long inhales and exhales as a way to cope with the sensation.

#BrilliantBIT

While annoying, B.H. contractions also have a benefit! They help strengthen your uterine muscles to prep for labor.[131] #gouterusgo!

#BrilliantTIP

Be sure to go to bed at a reasonable hour once you are at 37 weeks. You don't want the one day you stay up till 1 a.m. to be the day labor starts!

A CHANGE HAS OCCURRED!

Labor begins . . . dun dun dun

- Your water breaks. (See pg 108.)

- You start having wave-like, semi-consistent contractions.

OKAY, IT'S LABOR (aka Early Labor)

How long: Can last for a few hours to a few days. For many, it starts in the middle of night.

Physical Experience

- Contractions:

  - Irregular pattern with downtime between (could be seven minutes, ten minutes, twenty minutes, who knows!)

  - They're short! *Under* one minute each.

  - The sensations are manageable. You may be able to talk through them or you may need to pause momentarily, but they don't take everything you've got to make it through.

- You might have an urge to eat a big meal.

- You might feel nauseous and icky.

Emotional Experience

- You are still social, distractible.

- It may be hard to let yourself rest or go about your day because you feel anxious or excited or both that labor has begun. Remember to try and ignore your labor during this phase!

A CHANGE HAS OCCURRED!

Eek! These contractions are picking up.

- Contractions are starting to last longer, come closer together, and be more intense.

- A definite, consistent contraction pattern is starting to show itself.

- You need to pause to breathe through and cope with your contractions.

- You can't be as sociable anymore.

PHASE 2:

IS IT TIME TO GO YET? DOES THE MIDWIFE COME OVER?!
(aka transitioning to Active Labor)

How long: Lasts for hours, not days.

Physical Experience

o   Contractions: Clearly coming closer together, lasting longer, and feeling more intense.

o   Finding a comfortable position is hard.

o   Laying down is less comfortable.

o   You may feel nauseous.

o   You may vomit.

Emotional Experience

o   You don't want people talking to you during a contraction.

o   You need to focus to get through your contractions.

o   Shit . . . these are hard!

o   Is it time to go to my birthing place yet?

A CHANGE HAS OCCURRED!
It's likely "Active Labor"

At least two of the following are happening . . .

o   Contractions are coming every couple of minutes consistently, lasting for a *full minute* (fifty seconds doesn't count!) and this has been happening for *at least* a full hour.

o   You see bloody show—sort of like a period—not your mucus plug.

o   You feel rectal pressure—like you have to poop.

> ### #BrilliantTIP
> Remember that back labor (see pg 121) can mimic an active labor pattern of intense contractions and rectal pressure before you're clinically in active labor (5–6 cm). See pg 218 for tips to create space for baby to turn and pg 216 for support while in labor.

PHASE 3:

OMG, THESE CONTRACTIONS ARE INTENSE
(aka Officially Active Labor)

How long: Typically lasts for hours, in the single digits.

Physical Experience

All of the above, plus:

- You may vomit.
- You may feel nauseous.
- You may feel hot, then cold, then hot again, then cold . . .
- You may have the shakes.
- Clinically you're considered to be in active labor when you're 6 cm dilated.

> ### #BrilliantTIP
> This is typically a good time to go to your birthing place, ensure your midwife is at your home, or get an epidural if you are choosing one.

Emotional Experience

- You need to use your coping techniques—and your support team—to make it through the contractions.
- You might feel overwhelmed, scared, tired, and/or like labor sucks.
- You may be surprised by the sensations you are feeling—they are different than you expected!
- You may feel like finally you made it! Things are moving!

> **#BrilliantTIP**
>
> If at any point you feel like something is off, see green or brown in your fluids, or (and remember, this is very rare!) see excessive bleeding, feel stillness (you will likely feel your baby move less at this point—this is normal), or aren't sure, trust your Gut. Check in with your provider.

A CHANGE HAS OCCURRED!
I think I'm gonna poop my pants (nah, that's just baby)

- Feeling like you're going to poop yourself during contractions
- Making involuntary grunting sounds

- Shaking
- Sweating/feeling very hot
- I'm done! Give me that epi (if you don't have one yet)!

PHASE 4:
TRANSITIONING TO PUSHING

How long: Minutes to a few hours

Physical Experience

- Contractions:
  - Similar to active labor, but contractions are feeling even more intense and lasting a little bit longer: a bit over one minute each.

- Sweating
- Shaking
- An irresistible urge to push
- Vomiting
- More blood
- Involuntary grunting sounds

Emotional Experience

- Oh man, this is INTENSE!

- A feeling like you are so completely done and you want that epidural (if you don't have one).

A CHANGE HAS OCCURRED!

Now I really think I'm gonna poop

- The rectal pressure is constant and doesn't go away between contractions.

- You're pushing involuntarily.

- You're fully dilated!

PHASE 5:

PUSHING

The average for first-time pushers is *at least* two hours. If this isn't your first time, it may move more quickly. Regardless, we are talking a few hours in the single digits, tops.

➊ SNOOZE BREAK

HOW LONG: 10–30 min, or not at all

BODY: Some people experience this "resting phase" right before pushing. Though you are fully dilated, your contractions may slow down and space out.

EMOTIONS: You may feel energized, more aware of your surroundings, or perhaps scared of pushing. Take advantage of this period as much as you can. Rest up!

② PRAIRIE-DOGGING IT

HOW LONG: Minutes to a few hours

BODY: Remember that pubic bone? (See pg 84.) Well, getting baby's head to come down and under it is usually the longest phase of pushing. Baby's head has to "prairie-dog" it for a while, meaning the head comes down under the bone when you push, and then gets sucked back up as soon as you stop pushing. That bone is really in the way! While this can certaintly feel frustrating, it's good to remember that you are moving forward. Even though it can be a slow process, you are moving two steps forward and one step back until baby makes it past that pubic bone for good. It's typically smoother sailing from there.

EMOTIONS: Determination and also WTF?! Why is it taking so long?! Get outta there baby!

③ RING OF FIRE

HOW LONG: Minutes

BODY: You made it past the pubic bone! Yahoo! Next comes the sensation of your perineal area stretching as baby's head crowns. Remember the sensation is actually protective—it allows you to slowly stretch before baby's head plops out.

EMOTIONS: Holy shit. Holy shit. Holy shit.

④ HALF IN, HALF OUT

HOW LONG: Seconds to minutes

BODY: Generally, there's a brief break once baby's head makes it through—if you stare down between your legs, you'll literally see baby's head just chilling out there, but their body is still inside you! What a wild reminder that you are passing a human being through your body. Take it in! Baby's body generally slips out pretty quickly from here.

EMOTIONS: These are your final pushes, and they won't be nearly as intense as the ones that came before. You may feel excited to finally meet your baby, excited for it all to just be over, a little anxious that you're about to officially be a parent, and/or totally out of it and not very conscious of what you're feeling at all. When baby is born, some people are ready straightaway to bring their baby to their chest and snuggle, and other people need a second. You do you!

⑤ THE PLACENTA

HOW LONG: It typically takes between 5 and 45 minues before the placenta is ready to be born. Once it is, birthing it usually takes only a few minutes.

BODY: You will still feel contractions once baby is born (albeit they won't feel nearly as strong as labor contractions and you'll likely be quite distracted by your baby). For the most part, birthing the placenta is a pretty easy breezy process in comparison to every-thing else you just went through—remember placentas don't have bones! But sometimes, the placenta needs a little help being born. In this case your provider may need to put their hands inside of you to help the placenta detach and massage your uterus externally to help it contract. This kind of sucks, but usu-ally moves quickly. (Just a warning!) Once that placenta is born, you will feel the sweet, sweet relief of emptiness inside you.

EMOTIONS: OMG I had a baby!

CHEAT SHEET: COPING WITH LABOR

This list is meant to help you remember that you are never at a dead end in labor. There is always something else you can try. You'll likely need to experiment and play around to see what works best for you, but the possibilities are endless. And what helps at one point in your labor will likely change as labor changes—so just keep trying new things and return to your old tricks too in case they prove useful again later in your labor. This is a great page to share with your partner and support team.

Setting the Tone

PHYSICAL ENVIRONMENT

Goal: Making your physical space supportive of your labor

- The lighting—do you prefer them on, off, or dimmed?

- The vibes—would candles (battery operated if in a hospital), trinkets, photos, etc., be useful?

- The people—who is there with you?

- The location—do you need to change rooms? Go outside? Head to your birth place?

- Your body in your physical space— do you want your eyes open or closed? Are you comfortable in what you are wearing? Are there noises or talking that is distracting you?

ALL SYSTEMS GO

Goal: Making sure you are taking care of your physical body so that it can perform at its optimum.

- Pooping and peeing

- Eating and staying hydrated

- Resting

Staying in the Flow

DISTRACTIONS

Goal: Get yourself out of the "waiting" mindset, forget about the time, and try to ignore your labor for as long as you can. (Put that contraction timing app away!) This is especially good for pre-labor and early labor.

- Hang with friends
- Date nights
- Movies or TV
- Podcasts
- Play games
- Working
- Craft projects
- Baking
- *Grounding down* (see pg 153)

GO FROM REST PERIOD TO REST PERIOD.

Goal: Sleep when you can. Rest when you can't sleep. Make those *rest and recover* periods count (see pg 126). Try this in between contractions to help.

- Massage
- Tickles or gentle touch
- Scalp rub
- Soothing music or meditation tracks
- Resting positions (see pg 223)
- Get in the bath if your water hasn't broken yet.

RELEASE TO RESET.

Goal: When you feel overwhelmed, like your labor is stagnant, and/or you just wanna psych yourself up to get back in the game.

- Communicating how you are feeling
- Communicating your needs
- Screaming
- Crying
- Audible exhales
- Shaking it out
- Dancing
- Making weird, funny, nonsensical noises with your mouth—the weirder, the better.
- Stomping
- Orgasm
- Changing up your physical environment

OVERRIDE YOUR *PERSONAL SOUNDTRACK* BETWEEN CONTRACTIONS.

Goal: Helping your Head not freak out. You don't need to convince yourself to like labor. It's cool for you to hate it!

- Try to remind yourself that it is temporary and will be over soon enough.

- Remind yourself that people have been doing this for a long, long time! You aren't alone. Hello, Gut!

- Remind yourself you are capable and you *can* do it! Or repeat any other mantra or phrase that works for you (check your notes from part 1).

- *Drop in* to your Body.

- *Release to reset.*

- *Distractions*

- Listen to music.

- Listen to a meditation track.

STAY NICE AND OPEN.

Goal: Engage in movements and positions that keep the hips nice and open and baby moving down the canal in between contractions—and during when possible.

- Go on a walk.

- Positions to keep hips open (see pg 218)

- Walking up stairs two at a time

- Switch positions in bed if you are resting or have an epidural. (See pg 224.)

- Create more space in the hips if you are feeling back labor. (See pg 216.)

Coping with Strong Contractions

GO *WITH* THE CONTRACTIONS.

Goal: Letting your body lead. Sink into your contractions instead of fighting them. (Remember the visual on pg 126.)

- Dance or sway.

- Figure eight on a birth ball

- Long, deep inhales and exhales

- Stay in positions that keep your hips open (see pg 218) and either move in a downward motion with the contractions or breathe deeply in and out through them.

- Use your voice: humming, om-ing, chanting, singing, saying "yessss"—any sound that lets your vocal cords vibrate and welcomes the sensation.

- Nitrous oxide (if available)

OVERRIDE THE SENSATION.

Goal: Giving yourself something else to focus on instead of the sensations of the contraction.

- Get in the bath or shower.

- Pressure on the sacrum

- Hip squeeze (see pg 222)

- Heat or cold packs

- Use your voice (as above): Focus your attention on that vibrating sensation.

- Find a visual focal point and focus on it as you breathe deeply throughout the contraction.

- Smell an essential oil as you move through the contraction.

- Squeeze something with your hand—but make sure the squeezing is actually allowing the rest of your body to release.

- An epidural, if it is available and the right choice for you

TUNE OUT YOUR *PERSONAL SOUNDTRACK* DURING A CONTRACTION.

Goal: Getting out of that Head of yours when it tells you it hurts too much or that you can't do it.

- Sing a silly song quickly—in your head or out loud.
- Listen to music or a podcast you like.
- Count through the contraction.
- Repeat a mantra, phrase, or just keeping saying "yes."
- *Override the sensation* and focus on the new sensation or sense being activated.
- Listen to someone else's voice talk you through the contraction.

WHEN YOU HAVE BACK LABOR.

Goal: Creating more space in your hips for baby to renegotiate their positioning and help you release into the discomfort.

- Put a heat pack on the lower back.
- Get in a warm shower or bath if your water hasn't broken yet.
- Apply pressure to the sacrum.
- Do the exercises on pg 222.
- Squeeze hips during contractions.
- If you feel the urge to push but it isn't time to start pushing yet, getting on all fours can take some of the pressure off your back/butt.

DURING PUSHING

Goal: Helping you through the final push.

- Fresh smelling essential oils. We like eucalyptus, mint, or lemon. Sometimes there can be some strong smells during this phase so taking a whiff in between pushes is a great way to refresh and reenergize.

- Cold compress on the forehead or back of neck or a mini fan—it gets hot up in there.

- Eat and drink something with some sugar (fruit, juice, coconut water, honey sticks) to keep your energy up.

- Go with your Gut and Body, but let your clinical provider guide you when necessary. (See pg 149 for minimizing your risk of tearing.)

Using Your Compass

SELF CHECK-INS

Goal: Continuously checking in with yourself to see what you want and need, where you're stuck, and to remind yourself you are always moving forward!

- Going inward (see pg 100)
- Grounding down (see pg 153)
- Five-minute rule (see pg 140)
- Dropping in (see pg 20)
- Self-exam (see pg 120)

ADVOCATE.

Goal: Ensuring you stay an active participant in your labor and that things are happening *with* and *for* you, not *to* you.

- Stay home as long as you can if you are birthing in a hospital and you have no health indications to go in earlier.
- B.R.A.N.D. (see pg 139)
- *Five-minute rule* (see pg 140)

USE YOUR SUPPORT.

Goal: Remember you aren't in this alone! You have people—and your Baby!—to help you when you feel like you are suffering or stuck.

- Communicate when you need help or feel stuck, scared, anxious, etc., even if you aren't sure what you want or need.

- Let your support system help you with positions, massage, and touch, and be open to trying their suggestions—even if it sounds *terrible* at first, it may be just the thing.

- *Breathe with baby!* (See pg 16.)

POSITIONS TO OPEN THE PELVIS (Prepping for and during Labor)

Here are some tips and exercises to keep your pelvis open, your pelvic floor balanced, and to create more space in there for baby.

Before Labor

Things to do every day, everywhere . . .

- Keep your weight evenly distributed.
  - Try to avoid leaning on one hip while standing, sitting, or lifting.
  - Try not to favor a part of your feet—sides, heels, or balls.
- Lean forward, not back.

Stand up, put one hand on your tailbone and the other on your pubic bone, and lean forward. What do you feel happens? Now lean back. What do you feel happens? When you lean back, your pelvic outlet closes—and we want to keep it as open as we can.

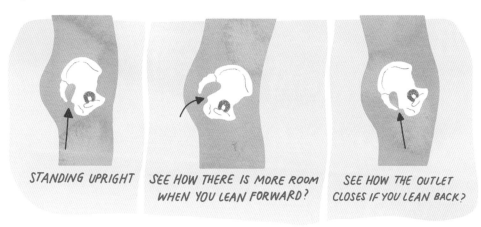

STANDING UPRIGHT   SEE HOW THERE IS MORE ROOM   SEE HOW THE OUTLET
WHEN YOU LEAN FORWARD?   CLOSES IF YOU LEAN BACK?

- ◉ Help yourself stay more forward by:
  - Supporting your back with pillows while sitting.
  - Hanging out on your birth ball as much as possible. (Bring one to work!)
  - Keeping your shoulders in front of your hips when laying on your side.
- ◉ Move a little every day.
- ◉ Exercising, going on walks, yoga, stretching, swimming, and using the stairs two at a time can all help you loosen things up and work with gravity to create more space.

And when possible:

- ◉ Call on your Body Squad (see pg 200)

During Labor

You always want to think: "downwards, open, and out!"

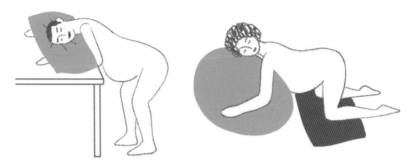

ALL FOURS. You can put pillows under your knees and do this on the floor, do it on your bed, or try it while supporting your upper body on top of a birthing ball. Try tucking and untucking your hips while you're there.

SITTING ON A BALL. Play some music and move your hips in exaggerated circles, or tilt the pelvis forward and back or side to side.

LEAN FORWARD. Stand, and then lean forward over any surface—stack pillows on said surface for comfort. Keep your knees slightly bent and spread your legs. This is great for resting and for contractions. During contractions, you can bend your knees and bring your butt down toward the floor or sway your hips from side to side.

#BrilliantTIP

Support people: Check their feet and shoulders. Often, when uncomfortable, our inclination is to bring our bodies upward instead of downward. Gently place a hand on their feet if they are standing on their toes or on their shoulders if you notice them creeping upward.

220

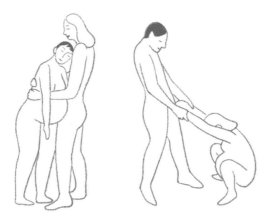

STAND AND HANG. Wrap your arms around a support person's neck, and let your body go. Or rest your head on their chest, freeing up your lower body. When a contraction comes, you can slow dance, bend those knees to bring your butt toward the ground or sway those hips in circles.

SUPPORTED SQUAT. Grab on to your support person or the frame of the bed.

#BrilliantTIP

Play around with the position of your feet. Try pointing your toes out and then in again. This will change which parts of your hips are opening!

LUNGE. Place one leg on a chair or couch and lunge into your lifted leg. Be sure your hips are squared out, they should not be squared toward your knee. Do both sides!

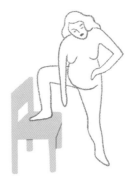

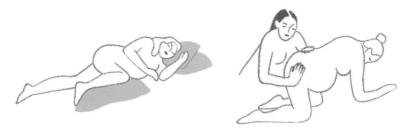

LAYING DOWN. Shift one leg all the way forward and the other all the way back. And always put pillows or a peanut ball in between your legs to keep those hips open. Switch sides every thirty minutes to one hour.

HIP SQUEEZE! Remember just how flexible that pelvis is? (See pg 82.) By applying pressure to the hips, you can actually create more space for baby—which means there is slightly less discomfort during the contractions. Support team take note: Be sure to check in to make sure you are applying the right amount of pressure. And, PSA: Once you're in position stay there until the contraction is over. Don't shift the pressure or remove your hands during the contraction unless they ask you too! Otherwise, you'll likely learn the hard way.

If You Have Back or Prodromal Labor

LIFT YOUR BELLY.

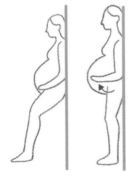

This does not feel good, but we've seen it do the trick! Stand against a wall, soften your knees, and tuck your pelvis forward so that your back is flat against the wall. When a contraction comes, lift your belly for the duration of the contraction. When it is over, let your belly go. Repeat this move for about ten contractions and check in to see if the sensation in your back has changed.

SPEND TIME ON ALL FOURS.

See pg 248 for more resources.

RESTING POSITIONS
(In Labor)

We know it can be hard to find a position to rest while in labor. Give these a try!

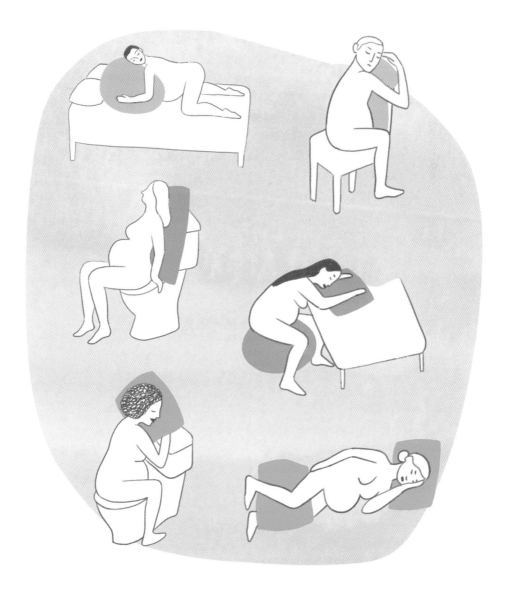

TOP TIPS FOR AN EPIDURAL

1. **Wait to get it until you need it.** This means either you are clinically in active labor (5–6 cm) or feeling enough discomfort or exhaustion that you are at your limit.

2. **Do the setup upon arrival.** If you know you are definitely getting an epidural or are likely going to want one at some point, get an IV upon arrival. They can't administer the epi unless you've had fluids, so this will help the process be quicker when you are ready. You can also sign the consent forms ahead of time.

3. **Ask who will actually be administering the epi.** Make sure you feel comfortable with the skill level and experience of that person. (It is possible for it to be a resident.) You can always ask for someone else.

4. **Sleep while you have it.**

5. **Use a peanut ball and change positions every thirty minutes or so.** See that red thing on the next page? That's a peanut ball. Google it, and buy one or check in with your hospital to see if they have them. This will help keep your hips open; we've seen it work wonders.

6. **Push that button.** Many hospitals nowadays utilize epidurals that have a self-dosing mechanism. This means that you can give yourself an extra dose of meds when you feel you need it. These are controlled so that you can't overdose. The whole point of the epi is to help you rest and to give you a break. So if you are uncomfortable enough that you are unable to do so, press that button.

7. **Be careful of "topping-off" before pushing.** In addition to self-dosing, it is also possible for the anesthesiologist to administer *more* medication through the epidural line. This is called a top-off. As your body gets ready to push, the contraction sensations can

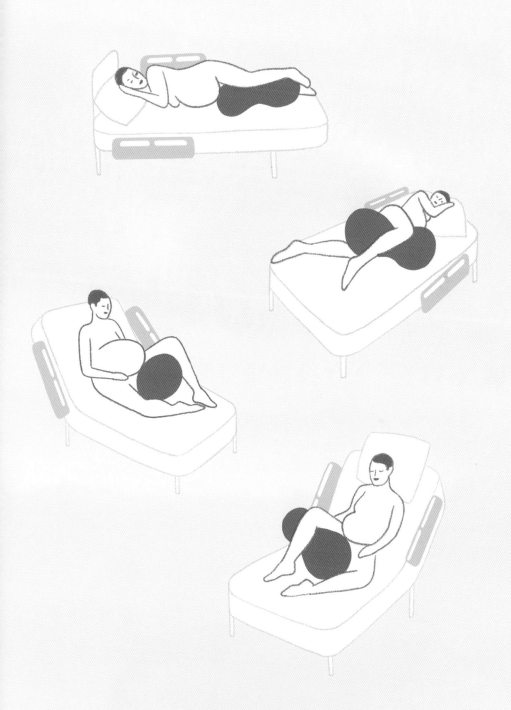

intensify. Even with the epidural, you may feel intense pressure in your butt or start to feel contraction sensations again—though it will not be as intense as pre-epi! It's common for well-intentioned doctors and nurses to offer you a top-off to make the sensations go away. However, this can make you extra numb. And the more numb you are, the harder it can be to push, so your risk of other interventions increases. Get a cervical exam to see where you are before agreeing to a top-off. It just might be time for you to start pushing—and being able to feel when you push can be a very good thing! If it is not time to push, getting a top-off may be a helpful tool.

8　**Epidurals can be turned off or lowered.** If you are having trouble pushing because you are numb, ask for your epi to be lowered or shut off. It takes a bit for it to wear off, so you won't go from 0 to 100, and it can make a big difference in how effectively you push.

9　**Speak up.** Because the staff assumes you are comfy with that epi, they may leave you for long stretches of time—although they are still monitoring your numbers on a screen outside. But remember, you have a ton of bodily information they don't have access to! If you feel pressure in your butt, are uncomfortable, in pain, feel contraction sensations on just one side, start feeling dizzy or light-headed, or at any point sense that something is just not right, listen to that Body and Gut and get the nurse.

A Few Notes on the Epidural Experience

The following aren't uncommon:

- **Uncontrollable shaking.** This will eventually go away. It is a side effect of the medication and also caused by your hormones.

- **Uncontrollable itching.** This will eventually go away. It is a side effect of the medication.

- **Your contractions stop or slow down.** You may need to get Pitocin to help bring them on again, or they may come back on their own.

- **You get a fever.**[132] While fever is a proven side effect of the epidural, it can also be a sign of infection. Because there is no way to know the definitive cause of a fever, you will likely be treated for infection, just in case. You may get antibiotics, and they may want to keep your baby overnight for observation.

- **Your blood pressure drops.**

- **You feel a lot of pressure still.** While the epi will take away the tightening and stretching sensations, it won't always take away the pressure you feel as baby's body descends through your pelvis.

- **You feel sensations on just one side.** If you feel your contractions mostly on one side, it could be because you've been laying on the other side for a long time. Gravity can make the epidural more concentrated on one half of your body. Be sure to check with your nurse/anesthesiologist and try turning to the other side to see if the medicine evens out.

- **You feel sweet, sweet relief.** Take advantage of it and rest up!

TOP TIPS FOR BREAST/CHEST-FEEDING

IT SHOULDN'T HURT.

This doesn't mean your nipples won't experience some wear and tear or you won't experience any discomfort. But you shouldn't be suffering, feeling sharp pains, seeing blood, or have cracked nipples. If this is you, get support ASAP. *Don't just push through and suffer through feedings.*

IT TAKES TIME!

It can take a while—we're talking over a month!—before you fully get the hang of breast/chest-feeding, because it is new for both you and baby. Just keep trying and ask for support throughout.

IT'S OKAY IF BREAST/CHEST-FEEDING ISN'T THE RIGHT CHOICE FOR YOU.

The benefits of breast/chest milk are real. But what is also real is your sanity, particularly during this time. There are many reasons why breast/chest-feeding may not be the best for you. You do you! And there's no need to defend your decision to anyone.

DON'T BE SO QUICK TO RESTRICT YOUR DIET.

There are no dietary restrictions when you are breast/chest-feeding, yahoo! (You should always check in about medications, herbs, and supplements, though.) It is very common for newborns to be gassy while their digestive systems are first learning how to work. This *does not mean* they are allergic to your milk! True allergies are very rare, so don't start putting new rules or restrictions on yourself unless your IBCLC feels it is necessary.

228

DRINK WATER ALL DAY EVERY DAY.

You lose water each time you feed or pump, so it is very important you stay super-hydrated. Your body is going to prioritize baby over you, meaning water goes to your milk before it goes to your body. So while it would take extreme dehydration to affect your supply, your body may feel the effects if you don't drink enough, in the form of dry skin, chapped lips, and less energy. Keep a water bottle with you always and try to drink about ten full glasses per day.

AIR-DRY.

As great as those nipple creams and pads can be, they can also hold on to *too much* moisture, allowing for yeast to grow. Air-dry your nips as often as you can! #freethenipple

SALINE SOAKS

This is our fave cure for sore or cracked nipples. Add one tablespoon of salt to warm water and let your nipples soak for a few minutes. It's a funny sight, we know! Repeat a few times throughout the day as needed. Air-dry.

FOR WHEN THEY ARE HARD AS A ROCK

Lots of massage from the armpit down. Try applying heat and cold packs and see which works best for you. If you have a pronounced lump, put an electric toothbrush or vibrator on the spot to loosen it up.

EMPTY THEM.

Okay, they'll never actually be "empty," but it is good to get used to feeding on each side until that breast/chest feels somewhat soft and empty. It will prevent issues like infections and plugged ducts and help your babe get the most of the milk.

KEEP THEM EVEN.

Remember each side has its own feedback loop, so keep track of which side you left off on, especially if you weren't able to get both sides in during one feeding sesh. PSA: It's normal if one side produces more than the other, so don't worry if you're lopsided—most people are! As long as there's no pain or other difficulties, it's probably a normal and common anatomical difference.

LEARN TO FEED WHILE LYING DOWN.

This will be a game changer for those long nights. Google "side-lying position" for a good visual on how to set it up.

AFTER A CESAREAN

You might have to get more creative with breast/chest-feeding positions to avoid putting weight or pressure on the scar. Putting a pillow over your lap to protect your scar can be helpful.

Introducing a Bottle

The recommendation is to wait to introduce a bottle or artificial nipples (like a pacifier) until breast/chest-feeding is well established to avoid nipple confusion or baby refusing the breast/chest because the bottle's flow is faster and easier. While this is different for everyone, generally a good time is at about 4–6 weeks. Whenever the right time is for you, check out *paced bottle-feeding* and other helpful resources on pg 248. Visit page 189 for tips before going back to work.

PUMPING TIPS

- **Check in with your insurance company.** They are required by law to provide you with a free pump. If you are pumping often, see if you can get a medical-grade one.

- **Pump innovation (finally)!** While many of these new pumps are not yet covered by insurance, if you are able and willing to pay, you do have options. Some are now noiseless, wireless, "smart pumps," superlightweight . . . do your research!

- **What about those manual pumps?** While we don't recommend *only* getting one of these since they get tiring, a manual pump can be good to have around for when you need a quick release but don't have time to do a full pumping sesh.

- **Make it hands-free!** Even if your pump requires your hands, you can get a pumping bra that makes it hands-free.

- **You don't *need* to pump.** There is no "right time" to start giving your babe the bottle. So unless you are having supply issues, or there is a specific date you know you need to be someplace and your baby will need a bottle, you don't have to pump until you are ready.

- **Pumping mimics the feedback loop.** So remember, the more you empty your breasts, the more you produce! It also means you need to be careful that you're not pumping *too much* if you are still regularly breast/chest-feeding. This can tell your body to make more than you need, leading to oversupply. Find more support on pg 168.

- **Keep that milk flowin'!** Using warm compresses before pumping and/or massaging from the armpit down to the nipple before and during pumping can help move milk from the ducts to the nipple.

- **You generally get the most milk in the early a.m.** That means between 1 and 6 a.m.

- **How much you pump is not an indication of how much your babe is getting.** Your baby will always be more efficient than your pump.

- **Power pump.** If you need to up your supply, you can try pumping for ten minutes, resting for ten minutes, and repeating for one hour or so. The idea here is to mimic what your babe would do if they were cluster feeding (see pg 169). Remember, the more you empty your breasts, the more milk you'll produce.

- **Experiment.** Things are constantly changing, so don't give up if something isn't working for you right away. It may actually work tomorrow or even in a few hours. You will eventually find what works for you . . . and then you may have to switch it up again. Hang in there!

231

TOP TIPS FOR YOUR POSTPARTUM BODY

Our biggest tip: The more you can take it easy and be patient with yourself to heal, the better off you'll be.

TAKING CARE OF YOUR PERINEUM

If you have a vaginal birth, your perineum will likely be sore for a little while. Regardless of your perineal condition, it's never a bad idea to help it heal.

Here's how:

- Take a sitz bath with herbs. (Google it!)

- Create "padsicles." In your final weeks of pregnancy, put some witch hazel on maxi pads with wings and keep them in the freezer. For the first few days postpartum, wear them in some disposable underwear (lovely, we know). Switch to ice packs if still needed after around day 3 as the astringent can get to be too much.

- Use a peri bottle or bidet. Wash yourself after you go to the bathroom to avoid infections, and keep things clean.

- Avoid penetration. Wait for the go-ahead from your provider that you are healing okay and—more importantly—until you feel ready!

DON'T FORGET YOUR BUTT.

Avoid constipation like the plague. While you may already have hemorrhoids (so sorry!) from pregnancy, ensuring you aren't straining while pooping can avoid making them worse or getting them in the first place. (Straining isn't great for your perineal healing either.)

Tush Tools

- Eat fiber-rich foods.

- Look into stool softeners and probiotics.

- Use a squatty potty to help you "flow" more easily.

- If you do have hemorrhoids, use witch hazel and do sitz baths to ease the discomfort.

PS: If you notice you are bleeding when you poop, let your provider know.

HEALING FROM A C-SECTION

There are some key differences in the postpartum experience when you have surgery, though every body is different. What we outline here will be more severe for some and more manageable for others:

- It is very normal to have uncontrollable shakes and swollen legs immediately post-surgery. It should stop in the first few hours, though it can take a bit longer for the swelling to go down. You will be given some special legwear that massages your legs to prevent clots while you're in the hospital.

- It might take a day or so before you can get out of bed, so you may not get that shower right away. Once you can get out of bed, though, it is very important to slowly start walking and being upright—if you wait too long, it will be harder later.

- Your movements will be limited. Bending down and getting in and out of the bed, a couch, or a chair may be difficult to do in the beginning. If you have another kid, it will be harder to carry them.

- If you were sutured with stitches, they will dissolve on their own. But if staples were used instead, you might have to go back to your doctor's office to have them removed.

- Keep an eye on your scar to ensure it is healing well and not infected. Ice packs can be helpful in the days after the surgery for swelling and discomfort.

> **#BrilliantTIP**
> Once your scar is healed and you get the go-ahead from your provider, scar tissue massage is an important tool to break up any adhesions at the scar site. (You don't want these to build up.) Make it part of your everyday self-care routine by doing it in the shower or before falling asleep. This ritual can actually be emotionally healing as well for processing your experience. The sooner you start, the fewer adhesions will be created, but it's never too late to work on an old wound. (Pun intended.)

Watch Yourself

If you are birthing outside of your home, you will likely not see your care provider again for six weeks postpartum. That's a whole lot of time for things to happen! And again, while the body wants to heal, sometimes it needs some extra help, and there's no shame in that—your body just totally marathoned it! If at any point you are experiencing pain, feel unsure, or just want to check in, *do it.* If you are birthing at home, you will likely have more consistent care from your provider postpartum, but you are still the only one with yourself 24/7. It's always good to be on the lookout and reach out to your midwife if something feels off.

Some postpartum red flags include:

- Blood clots coming out of your vagina that are bigger than a golf ball.
- Heavy bleeding—either the blood is soaking through one of those big pads in less than one hour or you won't stop bleeding.
- Blurry vision or a bad headache that's not going away.
- Fever or flu-like feelings.

Longer-term postpartum red flags—and likely an indication that a pelvic floor specialist would be helpful—include:

- Incontinence

- Pain during sex

- A feeling of heaviness or pressure in the vagina/rectum

- A bulge in the vagina or a feeling that something is loose down there

- Tailbone or pubic bone pain

- Overall pain in the nether regions more than six weeks since you have given birth

Makin' It Easier on Ya

CREATE "STATIONS." The goal here is to eliminate as many steps as possible. Even if you live in a small apartment, by the twelfth dirty diaper, even moving into the next room will feel like a lot. Set up a basket with diapers, changing pad/blanket, wet wipes, burping cloths, nipple cream, and some water and snacks for you. You can either set up a few of these around your home or make yours portable and bring it with you as you move about your day. Just be sure you are resting your "station" on a raised surface so that you're not constantly bending. Definitely keep one by your bedside for night changes so you don't have to get up!

BE HANDS-FREE. Set yourself up to be hands-free while still keeping baby happy, by keeping them close by. A wrap or baby carrier works great for this. You can even wear it inside as you go about your day! Consider a bouncer for when you want to take a shower.

TRY BELLY WRAPS. While this doesn't work for everyone, some people find having some belly support postpartum to be helpful and restabilizing. The only way to know if it works for you is to try it! No one kind of wrap is necessarily better than the others. You can purchase a Velcro one on Amazon or watch YouTube videos on how to tie a long scarf around you.

DON'T FREAK OUT IF . . .
QUELLING YOUR POSTPARTUM CONCERNS

- **You bleed for weeks.** You may bleed for up to six weeks or so after baby is born. (See pg 74 for more on why.) You may even see blood clots the size of a golf ball passing through your vagina (eek!). Crazily, this too is normal. Bigger than a golf ball? Bleeding through a heavy pad in less than an hour? Call your care provider.

- **Your body aches.** You just worked really hard, and depending upon the circumstances of your labor, may have some extra reasons to *feel it*. This is why it is so important to take it slow and give yourself time to heal. If you can sneak in an Epsom salts bath while your babe is sleeping, go for it.

- **It takes time to bond with baby.** Sometimes it can take a while, and that's okay! Maybe you had a traumatic birth or postpartum experience, maybe you had to be separated, or maybe you just need some more time. It's all good. Doing skin-to-skin time can help.

- **You don't want anyone else to touch your baby.** We feel you. Your baby has been only yours for about ten months, and it's hard to all of a sudden have to share. Keep them close for as long as you need to. Eventually you will be ready to hand them over.

- **You have night sweats.** Due to hormonal shifts some people experience intense night sweating and hot flashes during the first weeks postpartum. #funtimes

- **Your vision changes.** If you experienced vision changes during your pregnancy, they are likely to last for a while postpartum. It should improve over time, so don't get a new prescription just yet!

- **You lose a bunch of your hair.** You can thank your hormones for this one too. For some, this can be really dramatic, and for others, less so. It does grow back, but particularly for those really experiencing some bald spots, we know it's tough while it is happening. Hang in there and speak with a nutritionist and/or herbalist about how you can best supplement and support your body in the meantime.

- **Your feet are ginormous.** That's an exaggeration, but it is possible for your feet to get bigger and wider and stay that way post-pregnancy. That relaxin also relaxed your feet ligaments making your bones spread.

DON'T FREAK OUT IF . . .
WEIRD BABY STUFF THAT'S
TOTALLY NORMAL

When They Are First Born

- **They don't cry.** Sometimes babies come out a little shocked and need a second to know what to do. And once they do start crying, no need to stress over making them stop. Crying is actually a defense mechanism that helps babies clear the extra amniotic fluid often left behind in the lungs, thus allowing them to breathe more easily over time. So if they keep on wailin', it doesn't mean you're failin'!

- **They come out blue.** Babies don't use their lungs while in utero so they can be a little blue when they first come out. But don't worry: your baby won't look like a smurf forever. Usually within minutes they pink up, though their feet and hands may stay blue for longer since it takes a bit of time for the blood flow to reach the extremities.

237

- **Their head looks like a cucumber.** No, your babe is not an alien! If your child was birthed vaginally, it is common for the baby to have a cone head when they are born since their skull bones shifted to help them make it through the canal (see pg 94). It will get back into shape within a week or so.

- **Their body is covered in . . . cheese?!** Some babies are coated in a white cheese-like substance when they are born. This is called vernix, and it is how your baby's skin stayed protected while in utero. Think of it as their first moisturizer! It's not really cheese.

And in the First Few Weeks Baby . . .

- **Goes crossed-eyed.** Babies' eyes are not fully developed when they are born, so they wander and cross every so often. In fact, your babe won't be able to see colors or focus on anything farther than 8–10 inches away—which happens to be the distance to your face when you're feeding them!—until about 5–8 months.[133]

- **Sheds their skin.** If you were in a pool for ten months, your skin would shed too! There's no need to do anything here except avoid frequent baths, soaps, and perfumes.

- **Looks like they have bruises on their butt.** These bluish-gray spots are called Mongolian blue spots and are common birthmarks that typically appear on the lower back, but can be elsewhere on the body too. They tend to disappear over time.

- **Gets a bad case of acne.** About 20 percent of newborns get acne.[134] You can't do anything for it; it just goes away on its own. Expect to see it during the first six weeks and avoid using any products or treating it in any way, though you can try putting some breast/chest milk on it and see if it helps!

- **Has an icky belly button.** Even after the cord falls off completely—which tends to happen during the first 10–14 days—you might still see brown spots and even a little blood for a while longer. Check in with your pediatrician if you see any pus or signs of infection like excessive redness or a fever. Otherwise leave it alone and avoid putting rubbing alcohol on it.

○ **Bleeds from their vagina.** So strange we know, but about 3–5 percent of newborn babies have bloody discharge within the first five days after birth.[135] It is caused by a drop in the estrogen levels that were high while baby was still attached to the placenta. There's nothing to do here except don't freak out!

○ **Gets a boner!** It's a sign of a healthy nervous system and can also happen when their bladder is full.

○ **Has swollen breasts/genitals.** Due to extra hormones and extra fluid, it is possible for your baby's genitals and/or chest to appear swollen. It's also possible for whitish discharge to come out of their nipples. Just another thing we thought you should know. There's nothing to do here.

○ **Barfs like you did in college after a night out.** While it can look very dramatic, newborns spit and vomit. It's simply what they do. Usually this is not a reason for concern unless your baby seems to be in pain right before or after vomiting, which can be a sign of reflux. Check in with your doc if this is the case.

○ **Wants to be held 24/7.** That's how much they like you. But trust us, one day, your baby will walk away from you . . . and it might just break your heart a little. Remember, you can't spoil your baby!

○ **Looks like Wolfman.** Some babies are born with soft hairs all over their body—especially the shoulders, back, forehead, and cheeks. This is called lanugo, and it kept them warm in the uterus. It will fall out over time, so enjoy your fuzzy baby while you can.

○ **"Breathes" from their head.** Since babies are born with their skull bones not fused together yet, they have something called fontanelles, or spaces between the skull bones. It is common to see these fontanelles pulsing, especially the one at the top of their head. This just means there is blood flowing to your baby's brain. If you notice this soft spot is sunken, it can be a sign of dehydration, so call your pediatrician just in case.

PARTNERS, READ THIS PAGE

Dear partners,

First off, thank you for being here. Though it might feel like this "isn't about you," it really is—in a major way. It's so much harder to have to do this alone, and *you* can support your partner in ways that no one else can.

But it ain't easy.

So if you get nothing else from this book, we hope you can walk away with this: Transitions are hard, no matter how much grace we have as we move through them. And you too are going through a transition. You likely have your own slew of emotions, feelings, and fears coming to light. You may even feel an *added* pressure because you have to take care of your partner. You may feel like your feelings need to matter less right now because you aren't the one going through this huge physical experience. And maybe it feels like your partner is being unreasonable or crazy at times. And all the while your own needs are being ignored. It's a lot.

The physicality of pregnancy and birth is truly astronomical. (Please read pg 53.) And your partner is moving through a huge emotional transition while their Body is doing a lot of crazy shit—including upping their hormones to extreme levels so that your baby can grow and be healthy. So we ask this of you: just keep showing up. This doesn't mean that your needs should be ignored forever or that you can't express how you feel. In fact, it's just the opposite. Share how you feel as things come up, instead of letting those feelings turn into bitterness. And share from a place of wanting to connect *more* with your partner, instead of being reactive. Speak *of* your pain ("I am overwhelmed") so that you don't speak *from* your pain ("This sucks!"). Being aware of your own feelings will help you be present when your partner needs you the most. In fact, taking care of your own feelings *is* taking care of your partner.

And when your partner is killing you, err toward extreme patience and kindness instead of judgment. Give them the benefit of the doubt. Let your partner know they are safe to express their true needs.

If you're feeling like you don't know how you'll bond with this baby because you *aren't* having the physical experience, know that you can start building your own relationship with your babe in utero. (It might feel silly but see below!) And know that it's also okay to want to wait until you meet them.

We know all this is a bit abstract. So here are some specific reminders for you for the stages in the process in case they aren't obvious.

PRE-LABOR

- Speak to the babe in utero. They'll recognize your voice on the outside!

- Play or sing the same song for them over and over again in utero. They'll recognize it on the outside too!

- When your partner is at term (37 weeks), go to bed on the earlier side with them so that labor doesn't start when you are both exhausted.

- Help them keep their minds off of their impending labor and the "waiting" by planning date nights and other fun things to do together in the final weeks.

- Go to prenatal appointments when you can.

- Encourage them to rely on their *Dream Team*. Remind them it's a necessity, not a luxury.

IN LABOR

- That Coping Cheat Sheet on pg 212 is for you to help facilitate your partner.

- Stay off your phone.

- Help them stay distracted and ignore their labor for as long as you can.

- Try to keep your cool. If you're stressed or nervous, your partner will likely pick up on it!

- Help them advocate (see pg 217), and remind them to keep *going inward* (see pg 100).

- Don't make them feel gross for anything that comes out of their vagina—or butt.

- Don't complain about how tired you are.

- Don't eat in front of them.

- Don't talk to them *during* contractions; wait until it's done.

- Help others remember to hold off on questions, poking, and prodding while they are contracting.

- Stay close even if they don't want to be touched or talked to.

- Deal with logistics.

- Learn the hip squeeze. (See pg 222.)

- Let them know how powerful, awesome, and freaking loved they are. And do it again and again.

POSTPARTUM

- If on days 3–5 they are particularly emotional, remind them that this is because their mature milk is coming in.

- Make sure they have water and snacks while breast/chest-feeding.

- Take over baby duties when you can so they can get some rest.

- Learn a newborn calming tip (see pg 248) so you can have a special bonding activity with the baby.

- Do lots of skin-to-skin with your babe.

- Help them remember postpartum is temporary.

- Manage family members overstaying their welcome or making your partner stressed out—especially if they are yours!

- Still don't make them feel gross for anything that comes out of their vagina or butt.

- Still encourage them to rely on their *Dream Team*. Remind them it's a necessity, not a luxury.

- Still let them know how powerful, awesome, and freaking loved they are. And do it again and again and again. Actually, always do that!

They picked you to be their partner for a reason! You've totally got this.

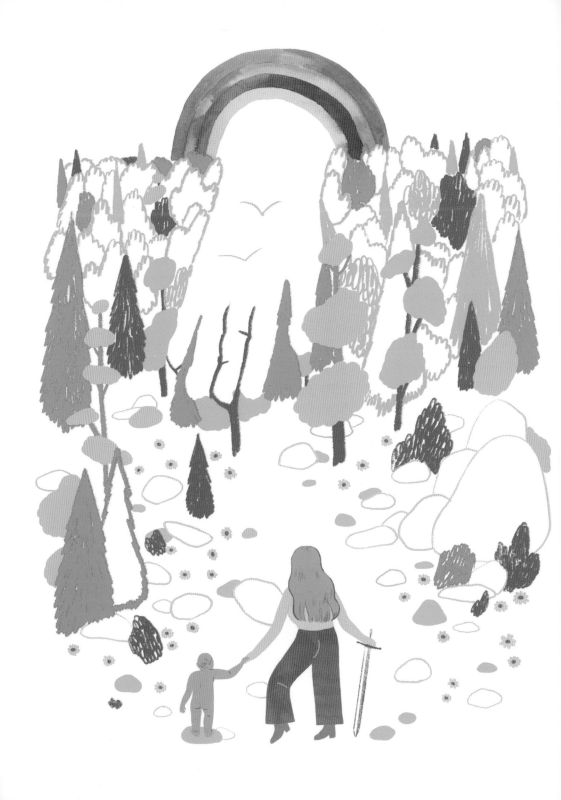

WE'LL LEAVE YOU WITH THIS . . .

BIRTH AS A LIFE METAPHOR: YOUR OWN POWER AS CREATOR

Holy moly.

Maybe now you can see why we think you are such a total badass—why we have lived on call for years, giving up family vacations and bar mitzvahs, showing up at the hospital with a little Halloween costume still stuck to our butts. Why we spent months and months and months pouring ourselves into this book so that we can start to shift how our culture approaches birthing.

Birth is a metaphor for *all* of our creative powers. It is a microcosm for every creative process—projects, art, businesses, new programs, new jobs. We are birthing stuff all the time whether we realize it or not. And there is *so much* we can learn from the process. So we hope that you can use this perinatal journey as an opportunity to discover and inspire awe over what *you,* as a creator, are capable of.

Remember, we *never* actually have control. We can *always* only *influence* and set the stage the best we can to succeed, with the best people to support us along the way. We *never* know the exact path, so we can *only* focus on how we move through it. And anytime we want to shift, to better ourselves, be bigger, we need to *go inward* along the way. We need to *tune in* to the compass inside of us. We need to contract in order to expand—hello, coping techniques!—because life is hard and scary at times, and there are growing pains we'll experience and lessons we need to learn along the way.

Our hope is that you now feel more confident in your power, in your unique tools, and your ability to navigate. Everything you learned here can also help you as you continue forging your path through parenthood and beyond.

Isn't it funny how loving our kids, our mini-mes, actually makes it easier to love and trust ourselves?

See: we weren't weren't kidding when we said all that growing can lead to incredible *growing*.

We're so freaking proud of you.

Onward!
Ash + Nat

Acknowledgments

How often do you get to write a book?! So we're really gonna go for the thank-yous here. Bear with us!

To the families that invited us into their lives: thank you. Doula work mirrors labor in so many ways—we too have to give up control, we don't know what the work will be like until we are in it, and we are forced to figure so much of it out on our own as we go along. Thank you so much for allowing us to be there. You are our greatest teachers.

And for those we couldn't help enough, let down, knew too little at the time, knew too much, left a lasting scar: please know we still hold you and we're *still* learning. We're sorry we couldn't be more for you at the time.

To all the badass midwives, doctors, childbirth educators, advocates, doulas, lawyers, practitioners, and community workers helping families have better perinatal experiences and to all those who paved the way before us: your words and influence likely made it into this book in one way, shape, or form. We are here because of you.

To the NYC Doula Collective: thank you for jump-starting our careers, for your mentorship and community. To Morgane and Alexandra: thank you for adding your voices here and for all the hard work you do for the LGBTQ+ community and beyond.

To our agent Giles, editor Shannon, art director Susan, and the whole Running Press team: thank you for taking a chance on us.

To Louise, the wonderous woman who filled these pages with such beautiful art and brought our concepts to life: we are beyond grateful.

To Chloe Campbell, CM, and Lucy French, CPM, LM for holding our information to the highest accuracy and making sure we didn't mess this up (special shout out to Lucy from Ash for being her *people*): thank you.

To Maya, Nat's little one. You show her the way. Your love is the best!

To our partners—you're our doulas!

And to our families, so much love. And deepest of gratitudes.

Resources

Our Fav Websites to Help You Navigate Your Health Care and Advocate for Yourself

● EVIDENCE BASED BIRTH

evidencebasedbirth.com

All the research you need to make informed decisions and have an educated convo with your provider around interventions, hospital policies, and more.

● CHILDBIRTH CONNECTION

childbirthconnection.org

Educational info to help you make informed choices and take care of your body during your pregnancy and postpartum period.

● MIDWIFE THINKING BLOG

midwifethinking.com

Learn about birth from a midwife and researcher's perspective.

● THE EDINBURGH POSTPARTUM DEPRESSION SCALE

fresno.ucsf.edu/pediatrics/downloads/edinburghscale.pdf

A self-assessment tool to check in on your mental health.

● ALLBODIES

allbodies.com

The hub for all things reproductive and sexual health. Learn about your body, purchase useful products to help you, and book appointments with practitioners who will actually listen to you!

Knowing and Protecting Your Rights

Rights As Breast/Chest-Feeding Person

● THE U.S. BREASTFEEDING COMMITTEE

usbreastfeeding.org/workplace-law

● NATIONAL CONFERENCE OF STATE LEGISLATURES—BREASTFEEDING STATE LAWS

ncsl.org/research/health/breastfeeding-state-laws.aspx

Protecting against Obstetric Violence

● BIRTH MONOPOLY

birthmonopoly.com

Adoption by LGBTQ+ Parents

● THE NATIONAL CENTER FOR LESBIAN RIGHTS

nclrights.org/wp-content/uploads/2013/07/2PA_state_list.pdf

Second-Parent Adoption

● HUMAN RIGHTS CAMPAIGN

hrc.org/resources/second-parent-adoption

Keeping Your Pelvis Nice and Open

● SPINNING BABIES
spinningbabies.com

● THE MILES CIRCUIT
milescircuit.com

Helping Your Baby Sleep

Safe Co-Sleeping Guidelines

● JAMES MCKENNA, the world's leading authority on mother*-infant co-sleeping in relationship to breastfeeding and SIDS
cosleeping.nd.edu/
safe-co-sleeping-guidelines

*language used by others

Caring for Your Baby at Night

● THE BABY FRIENDLY INITIATIVE (UNICEF)
unicef.org.uk/babyfriendly/
baby-friendly-resources/
sleep-and-night-time-resources/
caring-for-your-baby-at-night

Feeding Your Baby

● LA LECHE LEAGUE INTERNATIONAL
llli.org
Find local breast/chest-feeding support groups near you!

● KELLY MOM
kellymom.com
The bible for all things feeding your babe. Easy to navigate and answers to all your questions. Paced-bottle feeding, prepping a bottle, breast/chest-feeding concerns . . . they've got you.

● LACTMED DATABASE FOR MEDICATION SAFETY WHILE BREAST/CHEST-FEEDING
toxnet.nlm.nih.gov/newtoxnet/lactmed.htm
Find out which meds are safe to take while pregnant or breast/chest-feeding. Also a handy app!

Storing and Prepping Bottles
(breast/chest milk + formula)

● todaysparent.com/wp-content/
uploads/2016/08/
Breastmilk_Formula-Charticle.jpg

Watch These Videos!

A Correct Latch

● STANFORD MEDICINE
med.stanford.edu/newborns/
professional-education/breastfeeding/
a-perfect-latch.html

Breast/Chest-Feeding Positions

● med.stanford.edu/newborns/
professional-education/breastfeeding.html

Hand Expression

● med.stanford.edu/newborns/
professional-education/breastfeeding/
hand-expressing-milk.html

Perineal Massage

● mamanatural.com/perineal-massage/

Healing a C-Section Scar

● functionalpelvis.com/essential-free-
education

Important Reads

- *The Birth Partner: A Complete Guide to Childbirth for Dads, Doulas, and All Other Labor Companions* by Penny Simkin

- *Expecting Better: Why the Conventional Pregnancy Wisdom Is Wrong—and What You Really Need to Know* by Emily Oster

- *Gentle Birth, Gentle Mothering: A Doctor's Guide to Natural Childbirth and Gentle Early Parenting Choices* by Dr. Sarah Buckley and Ina May Gaskin

- *The Happiest Baby on the Block, Fully Revised and Updated Second Edition: The New Way to Calm Crying and Help Your Newborn Baby Sleep Longer* by Dr. Harvey Karp

- *Ina May's Guide to Childbirth* by Ina May Gaskin

- *Killing the Black Body: Race, Reproduction, and the Meaning of Liberty* by Dorothy Roberts

- *Lying In: A History of Childbirth in America* by Richard W. Wertz and Dorothy C. Wertz

- *Medical Apartheid: The Dark History of Medical Experimentation on Black Americans from Colonial Times to the Present* by Harriet A. Washington

- *Medical Bondage: Race, Gender, and the Origins of American Gynecology* by Deirdre Cooper Owens

- *Natural Health after Birth: The Complete Guide to Postpartum Wellness* by Aviva Jill Romm

- *This Isn't What I Expected: Overcoming Postpartum Depression* by Karen R. Kleiman, MSW, LCSW and Valerie Davis Raskin, MD

Important Films

- *The Business of Being Born*
An exploration of the maternity care system in America

- *Freedom for Birth*
Examining the issue of human rights in childbirth

- *MicroBirth*
An exploration of how the way babies are born is linked with health later in life.

- *Orgasmic Birth*
Documenting how birth can be pleasurable

250

Citations

1 Bohren MA1, Hofmeyr GJ, Sakala C, Fukuzawa RK, Cuthbert A. "Continuous support for women during childbirth." Cochrane Database Syst Rev. 2017 Jul 6;7:CD003766. doi:10.1002/14651858. CD003766.pub6.

2 WHO Reproductive Health Library. "WHO recommendation on daily fetal movement counting." (December 2016). The WHO Reproductive Health Library; Geneva: World Health Organization.

3 Alison Young, 2019. "Deadly deliveries: How hospitals are failing mothers," *USA TODAY*, March 6, 2019. https://www.usatoday.com/deadly-deliveries/interactive/how-hospitals-are-failing-new-moms-in-graphics/re fa.

4 Creanga, A.A., Syverson, C., Seek, K., & Callaghan, W.M. (2017). "Pregnancy-Related Mortality in the United States, 2011–2013." *Obstetrics & Gynecology*, 130(2), 366–373. doi: 10.1097/AOG.0000000000002114.

5 Rachel Reed, Rachael Sharman, and Christian Inglis. "Women's descriptions of childbirth trauma relating to care provider actions and interactions." *BMC Pregnancy and Childbirth*. (2017) 17:21. doi: 10.1186/s12884-016-1197-0.

6 Kertscher, Tom. "Americans Spend the Most on Health Care, Get Worst Outcomes?" PolitiFact. March 18, 2019. Accessed July 12, 2019. https://www.politifact.com/truth-o-meter/statements/2019/mar/18/tulsi-gabbard/yes-americans-spend-ton-health-care-worst-outcomes/.

7 Loudon, Irvine. *Death in Childbirth: An International Study of Maternal Care and Maternal Mortality, 1800–1950*. Oxford: Clarendon Press, 2001.

8 Judith Walzer Leavitt. *Brought to Bed: Childbearing in America 1750–1950*. New York: Oxford University Press, 1986.

9 Loudon, Irvine. *Death in Childbirth: An International Study of Maternal Care and Maternal Mortality, 1800–1950*. Oxford: Clarendon Press, 2001.

10 Benia, Cooper Owens Deirdre. *Medical Bondage: Race, Gender, and the Origins of American Gynecology*. Athens: University of Georgia Press, 2018.

11 Wertz, Richard W., and Dorothy C. Wertz. *Lying-in: A History of Childbirth in America*. New York: Free Press, 1990.

12 Wertz, Richard W., and Dorothy C. Wertz. *Lying-in: A History of Childbirth in America*. New York: Free Press, 1990.

13 Oparah, Julia Chinyere, and Alicia D. Bonaparte. *Birthing Justice: Black Women, Pregnancy, and Childbirth*. London: Routledge, Taylor & Francis, 2016.

14 Neal Devitt BA (1979). "The Statistical Case for the Elimination of the Midwife." *Women & and Health*, 4:1, 81-96. doi: 10.1300/J013v04n01_05 (1979z), 89.

15 Loudon, Irvine. *Death in Childbirth: An International Study of Maternal Care and Maternal Mortality, 1800–1950*. Oxford: Clarendon Press, 2001.

16 Nancy Langston, "The Retreat from Precaution: Regulating Diethylstilbestrol (DES), Endocrine Disruptors, and Environmental Health," *Environmental History* 13 (January 2008): 41–65.

17 Olsen O, Clausen JA. "Planned hospital birth versus planned home birth." Cochrane Database of Systematic Reviews 2012, Issue 9. Art. No.: CD000352. doi: 10.1002/14651858. CD000352.pub2.

18 Frank A. Chervenak, MDa, Laurence B. McCullough, PhDb, Robert L. Brent, MD, PhD, DSc (Hon)a,c, Malcolm I. Levene, MD, FRCP, FRCPH, F Med Scd, Birgit Arabin, MDe. "Planned home birth: the professional responsibility response." *American Journal of Obstetrics & Gynecology.* January 2013 Volume 208, Issue 1, Pages 31–38. doi: https://doi.org/10.1016/j.ajog.2012.10.002.

19 Vedam S, Stoll K, MacDorman M, Declercq E, Cramer R, Cheyney M, et al. (2018) "Mapping integration of midwives across the United States: Impact on access, equity, and outcomes." PLoS ONE 13(2): e0192523. https://doi.org/10.1371/journal.pone.0192523.

20 World Health Organization, 2015. "WHO Statement on Caesarean Section Rates." WHO/RHR/15.02 https://www.who.int/reproductivehealth/publications/maternal_perinatal_health/cs-statement/en/.

21 Eugene R. Declercq, PhD, Carol Sakala, PhD, MSPH, Maureen P. Corry, MPH, Sandra Applebaum, MS, and Ariel Herrlich, MA. "Major Survey Findings of Listening to Mothers III: Pregnancy and Birth Report of the Third National U.S. Survey of Women's Childbearing Experiences." *J Perinat Educ.* 2014 Winter; 23(1): 9–16. doi: 10.1891/1058-1243.23.1.9.

22 It's likely that the nongestational parent will not be able to access insurance-related information until the gestational parent signs paperwork to allow this. Be prepared to request this paperwork during some of the first interactions with the health insurance company.

23 Ina May Gaskin, 2003. *Ina May's Guide To Childbirth.* Bantam Books, 2008.

24 Hytten, Frank. "Blood Volume Changes in Normal Pregnancy." *Obstetrical & Gynecological Survey* 41, no. 7 (1986): 426–28.

25 Brewer, Sarah. *The Pregnant Body Book.* New York: DK Publishing, 2011.

26 Ramsey, E.M. (1994) "Anatomy of the human uterus." In Chard, T. and Grudzinskas, J.G. (eds), *The Uterus.* Cambridge University Press, Cambridge, pp. 18–40.

27 Surabhi Chandra, Anil Kumar Tripathi, Sanjay Mishra, Mohammad Amzarul, and Arvind Kumar Vaish. "Physiological Changes in Hematological Parameters During Pregnancy." *Indian J Hematol Blood Transfus.* 2012 Sep; 28(3): 144–146. doi: 10.1007/s12288-012-0175-6

28 Buckley, Sarah J. "Hormonal Physiology of Childbearing: Evidence and Implications for Women, Babies, and Maternity Care." Washington, D.C.: Childbirth Connection Programs, National Partnership for Women & Families, January 2015.

29 Gintzler, A.R., & Liu, N.J. (2001). "The maternal spinal cord: Biochemical and physiological correlates of steroid-activated antinociceptive processes." *Prog Brain Res*, 133, 83–97.

30 Mesiano S. The Endocrinology of Parturition. Basic Science and Clinical Application. *Front Horm Res.* Basel, Karger, 2001, vol 27, pp. 86–104. https://doi.org/10.1159/000061038.

31 Buckley, Sarah J. "Hormonal Physiology of Childbearing: Evidence and Implications for Women, Babies, and Maternity Care." Washington, D.C.: Childbirth Connection Programs, National Partnership for Women & Families, January 2015.

32 Khan, A.H., Carson, R.J., & Nelson, S.M. (2008). "Prostaglandins in labor—a translational approach." *Front Biosci*, 13(15), 5794–5809.

33 Russell JA, Douglas AJ, Ingram CD. "Brain preparations for maternity-adaptive changes in behavioral and neuroendocrine systems during pregnancy and lactation. And overview." *Prog Brain Res.* 2001;133:1-38.

34 Khan, A.H., Carson, R.J., & Nelson, S.M. (2008). "Prostaglandins in labor—a translational approach." *Front Biosci*, 13(15), 5794–5809.

35 Khan, A.H., Carson, R.J., & Nelson, S.M. (2008). "Prostaglandins in labor—a translational approach." *Front Biosci*, 13(15), 5794–5809.

36 Bendvold, E., Gottlieb, C., Svanborg, K., Bygdeman, M., & Eneroth, P. (1987). "Concentration of prostaglandins in seminal fluid of fertile men." *Int J Androl*, 10(2), 463–469.

37 Uvnäs-Moberg, K., Widström, A.M., Werner, S., et al. (1990). "Oxytocin and prolactin levels in breastfeeding women. Correlation with milk yield and duration of breast-feeding." *Acta Obstet Gynecol Scand*, 69(4), 301–306.

38 Nissen, E., Lilja, G., Widstrom, A.M., et al. (1995). "Elevation of oxytocin levels early post partum in women." *Acta Obstet Gynecol Scand*, 74(7), 530–533.

39 Faxelius, G., Hagnevik, K., Lagercrantz, H., et al. (1983). "Catecholamine surge and lung function after delivery." *Arch Dis Child*, 58(4), 262–266.

40 Nissen, E., Gustavsson, P., Widstrom, A.M., et al. (1998). "Oxytocin, prolactin, milk production and their relationship with personality traits in women after vaginal delivery or cesarean section." *J Psychosom Obstet Gynaecol*, 19(1), 49–58.

41 Sauriyal, D.S., Jaggi, A.S., & Singh, N. (2011). "Extending pharmacological spectrum of opioids beyond analgesia: Multifunctional aspects in different pathophysiological states." *Neuropeptides*, 45(3), 175–188.

42 Tornetta, G. (1998). *Painless childbirth: An empowering journey through pregnancy and childbirth.* Nashville TN: Cumberland House Publishing.

43 Buckley, Sarah J. "Hormonal Physiology of Childbearing: Evidence and Implications for Women, Babies, and Maternity Care." Washington, D.C.: Childbirth Connection Programs, National Partnership for Women & Families, January 2015.

44 Franceschini, R., Venturini, P.L., Cataldi, A., et al. (1989). "Plasma beta-endorphin concentrations during suckling in lactating women." *Br J Obstet Gynaecol, 96*(6), 711–713; Voogt, J.L., Lee, Y., Yang, S., et al. (2001). "Regulation of prolactin secretion during pregnancy and lactation." *Prog Brain Res, 133*, 173–185.

45 Zanardo, V., Nicolussi, S., Giacomin, C., et al. (2001). "Labor pain effects on colostral milk beta-endorphin concentrations of lactating mothers." *Biol Neonate, 79*(2), 87–90; Zanardo, V., Nicolussi, S., Carlo, G., et al. (2001). "Beta endorphin concentrations in human milk." *J Pediatr Gastroenterol Nutr, 33*(2), 160–164.

46 Varrassi, G., Bazzano, C., & Edwards, W.T. (1989). "Effects of physical activity on maternal plasma betaendorphin levels and perception of labor pain." *Am J Obstet Gynecol, 160*(3), 707–712; McMurray, R.G., Berry, M.J., & Katz, V. (1990). "The beta-endorphin responses of pregnant women during aerobic exercise in the water." *Med Sci Sports Exerc, 22*(3), 298–303.

47 Gaskin, I.M. (2003). "Going backwards: The concept of 'pasmo'." *Pract Midwife, 6*(8), 34–37.

48 Odent, M. (1987). "The fetus ejection reflex." *Birth*, 14(2), 104–105.

49 Neumark, J., Hammerle, A.F., & Biegelmayer, C. (1985). "Effects of epidural analgesia on plasma catecholamines and cortisol in parturition." *Acta Anaesthesiol Scand*, 29(6), 555–559.

50 Brewer, Sarah. *The Pregnant Body Book:*. New York: DK Publishing, 2011.

51 MacLennan AH. "The role of the hormone relaxin in human reproduction and pelvic girdle relaxation." *Scand J Rheumatol Suppl.* 1991;88:7-15.

52 Grattan, D.R., & Kokay, I.C. (2008). "Prolactin: A pleiotropic neuroendocrine hormone." *J Neuroendocrinol, 20*(6), 752–763.

53 Buckley, Sarah J. "Hormonal Physiology of Childbearing: Evidence and Implications for Women, Babies, and Maternity Care." Washington, D.C.: Childbirth Connection Programs, National Partnership for Women & Families, January 2015.

54 Nissen, E., Gustavsson, P., Widstrom, A.M., et al. (1998). "Oxytocin, prolactin, milk production and their relationship with personality traits in women after vaginal delivery or cesarean section." *J Psychosom Obstet Gynaecol,* 19(1), 49–58.

55 Emilie C. Rijnink, Marlies E. Penning, Ron Wolterbeek, Suzanne Wilhelmus, Malu Zandbergen, Sjoerd G. van Duinen, Joke Schutte, Jan A. Bruijn, Ingeborg M. Bajema. "Tissue microchimerism is increased during pregnancy: a human autopsy study." *MHR: Basic science of reproductive medicine*, Volume 21, Issue 11, November 2015, Pages 857–864, https://doi.org/10.1093/molehr/gav047; Amy M. Boddy, Angelo Fortunato, Melissa Wilson Sayres, Athena Aktipis. "Fetal microchimerism and maternal health: A review and evolutionary analysis of cooperation and conflict beyond the womb." *BioEssays*, 28 August 2015. https://doi.org/10.1002/bies.201500059.

56 "Delayed umbilical cord clamping after birth." Committee Opinion No. 684. American College of Obstetricians and Gynecologists. *Obstet Gynecol* 2017;129:e5–10; American College of Nurse Midwives. "Delayed umbilical cord clamping." Position Statement. Silver Spring (MD): ACNM; 2014. Available at: http://www.midwife.org/ACNM/files/ACNMLibraryData/UPLOADFILENAME/000000000290/Delayed-Umbilical-Cord-Clamping-May-2014.pdf. Retrieved September 1, 2016.

57 McDonald SJ, Middleton P, Dowswell T, Morris PS. "Effect of timing of umbilical cord clamping of term infants on maternal and neonatal outcomes." Cochrane Database of Systematic Reviews. 2013, Issue 7. Art. No.: CD004074. DOI: 10.1002/14651858.CD004074.pub3.

58 Morarji Peesay. "Cord around the neck syndrome." *BMC Pregnancy Childbirth*. 2012; 12(Suppl 1): A6. doi: 10.1186/1471-2393-12-S1-A6.

59 Kitzinger, S., *The Year After Childbirth*. New York: Charles Scribner, 1994.

60 Blanks, A.M., & Thornton, S. (2003). "The role of oxytocin in parturition." *BJOG, 110 Suppl 20*, 46-51; Fuchs, A.R., & Fuchs, F. (1984). "Endocrinology of human parturition: A review." *Br J Obstet Gynaecol,* 91(10), 948-967; Vrachnis, N., Malamas, F.M., Sifakis, S., et al. (2011). "The oxytocin-oxytocin receptor system and its antagonists as tocolytic agents" *Int J Endocrinol, 2011*, 350546.

61 Lagercrantz, H. (2016) "The good stress of being born." *Acta Paediatr*, 105: 1413–1416. doi:10.1111/apa.13615; Hillman, N.H., Kallapur, S.G., & Jobe, A.H. (2012). "Physiology of transition from intrauterine to extra-uterine life." *Clin Perinatol, 39*(4), 769–783.

62 Andreas NJ, Kampmann B, Le-Doare KM (2015). "Human breast milk: A review on its composition and bioactivity." *Early Human Development*, 91(11), 629–35.

63 Natalie Shenker MRSB. "The mysteries of milk." *The Biologist*. 64(3) p10-13. https://thebiologist.rsb.org.uk/biologist/158-biologist/features/1758-the-mysteries-of-milk.

64 Foteini Kakulas. "Protective Cells in Breast Milk: For the Infant and the Mother?" SPLASH! milk science update: APRIL 2013 Issue. https://milkgenomics.org/article/protective-cells-in-breast-milk-for-the-infant-and-the-mother/.

65 Iverson, S J. and O.T. Oftedal. 1995. "Phylogenetic and ecological variation in the fatty acid composition of milks." R.G. Jensen, ed., *The Handbook of Milk Composition*. Academic Press, Inc., Orlando. 789-–827.

66 Davis, Jasmine C. C., Zachery T. Lewis, Sridevi Krishnan, Robin M. Bernstein, Sophie E. Moore, Andrew M. Prentice, David A. Mills, Carlito B. Lebrilla, and Angela M. Zivkovic. "Growth and Morbidity of Gambian Infants Are Influenced by Maternal Milk Oligosaccharides and Infant Gut Microbiota." *Scientific Reports* 7, no. 1 (2017). doi:10.1038/srep40466.

67 Angela Garbes. 2015. "The More I Learn About Breast Milk, the More Amazed I Am." *The Stranger*, August 26, 2015. https://www.thestranger.com/features/feature/2015/08/26/22755273/the-more-i-learn-about-breast-milk-the-more-amazed-i-am.

68 Prentice AM, Prentice A (1988) "Energy costs of lactation." *Ann. Rev. Nutr.* 8:63-79. DOI: 10.1146/annurev.nu.08.070188.000431.

69 Geddes, Donna T., et al. "Tongue movement and intra-oral vacuum of term infants during breastfeeding and feeding from an experimental teat that released milk under vacuum only." *Early human development* 88.6 (2012): 443–449; Ramsay, D. T., Kent, J. C., Owens, R. A., & Hartmann, P. E. (2004). "Ultrasound imaging of milk ejection in the breast of lactating women." *Pediatrics*, 113(2), 361–367.

70 Al-Shehri SS, Knox CL, Liley HG, Cowley DM, Wright JR, Henman MG, et al. (2015) "Breastmilk-Saliva Interactions Boost Innate Immunity by Regulating the Oral Microbiome in Early Infancy." PLoS ONE 10(9): e0135047. https://doi.org/10.1371/journal.pone.0135047.

71 Cox DB, Owens RA, Hartmann PE. "Blood and milk prolactin and the rate of milk synthesis in women." *Exp Physiol*. 1996 Nov;81(6):1007–20; Kelly Bonyata, BS, IBCLC, 2018. "How does milk production work?" Updated on March 8, 2018. https://kellymom.com/hot-topics/milkproduction/.

72 Mahmood U, O'Donoghue K. "Microchimeric fetal cells play a role in maternal wound healing after pregnancy." *Chimerism*. 2014;5(2):40–52.

73 Gordon C.S. Smith. "Use of time to event analysis to estimate the normal duration of human pregnancy." *Human Reproduction*, Volume 16, Issue 7, July 2001, Pages 1497–1500, https://doi.org/10.1093/humrep/16.7.1497.

74 Eugene R. Declercq, PhD, Carol Sakala, PhD, MSPH, Maureen P. Corry, MPH, Sandra Applebaum, MS, and Ariel Herrlich, MA. "Major Survey Findings of Listening to Mothers III: Pregnancy and Birth. Report of the Third National U.S. Survey of Women's Childbearing Experiences." *J Perinat Educ*. 2014 Winter; 23(1): 9–16. doi: 10.1891/1058-1243.23.1.9.

75 Rebecca L. Dekker, PhD, RN, APRN. 2012. "What is the Evidence for Induction for Low Amniotic Fluid in a Healthy Pregnancy?" August 30, 2012 https://www.lamaze.org/Connecting-the-Dots/what-is-the-evidence-for-induction-for-low-amniotic-fluid-in-a-healthy-pregnancy.

76 https://evidencebasedbirth.com/evidence-on-inducing-labor-for-going-past-your-due-date/.

77 Rebecca L. Dekker, PhD, RN, APRN. 2016. "What is the Evidence on: Induction or C-section for a Big Baby?" Published in 2013 and updated on June 8, 2016. https://evidencebasedbirth.com/evidence-for-induction-or-c-section-for-big-baby/.

78 Eugene R. Declercq, PhD, Carol Sakala, PhD, MSPH, Maureen P. Corry, MPH, Sandra Applebaum, MS, and Ariel Herrlich, MA. "Major Survey Findings of Listening to Mothers III: Pregnancy and Birth. Report of the Third National U.S. Survey of Women's Childbearing Experiences." *J Perinat Educ*. 2014 Winter; 23(1): 9–16. doi: 10.1891/1058-1243.23.1.9.

79 Rebecca L. Dekker, PhD, RN, APRN. 2016. "What is the Evidence on: Induction or C-section for a Big Baby?" Published in 2013 and updated on June 8, 2016. https://evidencebasedbirth.com/evidence-for-induction-or-c-section-for-big-baby/.

80 Rebecca L. Dekker, PhD, RN, APRN. 2019. "Evidence on: Induction for Gestational Diabetes." Originally published on July 3, 2012 and updated on April 3, 2019. https://evidencebasedbirth.com/evidence-on-induction-for-gestational-diabetes/.

81 Gunn, G. C., Mishell, D. R., Jr., & Morton, D. G. (1970). "Premature rupture of the fetal membranes. A review." *Am J Obstet Gynecol*, 106(3), 469–483.

82 https://www.cdc.gov/groupbstrep/about/fast-facts.html.

83 Rebecca L. Dekker, PhD, RN, APRN. 2017. "Evidence on: Premature Rupture of Membranes." Originally published on November 20, 2014 and updated on July 10, 2017. https://evidencebasedbirth.com/evidence-inducing-labor-water-breaks-term/.

84 Marian F. MacDorman, Ph.D.; T.J. Mathews, M.S.; and Eugene Declercq, Ph.D. "Trends in Out-of-Hospital Births in the United States, 1990–2012." NCHS Data Brief No. 144, March, 2014 https://www.cdc.gov/nchs/products/databriefs/db144.htm.

85 Practice Bulletin No. 173: Fetal Macrosomia. *Obstet Gynecol.* 2016 Nov;128(5):e195-e209. American College of Obstetricians and Gynecologists' Committee on Practice Bulletins—Obstetrics.

86 Eugene R. Declercq, PhD, Carol Sakala, PhD, MSPH, Maureen P. Corry, MPH, Sandra Applebaum, MS, and Ariel Herrlich, MA. "Major Survey Findings of Listening to Mothers III: Pregnancy and Birth. Report of the Third National U.S. Survey of Women's Childbearing Experiences." *J Perinat Educ.* 2014 Winter; 23(1): 9–16. doi: 10.1891/1058-1243.23.1.

87 Eugene R. Declercq, PhD, Carol Sakala, PhD, MSPH, Maureen P. Corry, MPH, Sandra Applebaum, MS, and Ariel Herrlich, MA. "Major Survey Findings of Listening to Mothers III: Pregnancy and Birth. Report of the Third National U.S. Survey of Women's Childbearing Experiences." *J Perinat Educ.* 2014 Winter; 23(1): 9–16. doi: 10.1891/1058-1243.23.1.9.

88 "Safe prevention of the primary cesarean delivery." Obstetric Care Consensus No. 1. American College of Obstetricians and Gynecologists. *Obstet Gynecol* 2014;123:693–711.

89 "Shoulder dystocia." Practice Bulletin No. 178. American College of Obstetricians and Gynecologists. *Obstet Gynecol* 2017;129:e123–33.

90 Rouse DJ, Owen J, Goldenberg RL, Cliver SP. "The effectiveness and costs of elective cesarean delivery for fetal macrosomia diagnosed by ultrasound." *JAMA.* 1996 Nov 13;276(18):1480–6.

91 Morrison JC, Sanders JR, Magann EF, Wiser WL. "The diagnosis and management of dystocia of the shoulder." *Surg Gynecol Obstet.* 1992 Dec;175(6):515–22.

92 Kelly Milotay, 2013. "Cephalopelvic Disproportion (CPD)" July 24, 2013. http://www.ican-online.org/wp-content/uploads/2014/01/Question-CPD.pdf.

93 "Safe prevention of the primary cesarean delivery." Obstetric Care Consensus No. 1. American College of Obstetricians and Gynecologists. *Obstet Gynecol* 2014;123:693–711.

94 "Safe prevention of the primary cesarean delivery." Obstetric Care Consensus No. 1. American College of Obstetricians and Gynecologists. *Obstet Gynecol* 2014;123:693–711.

95 Michael C. Klein, MD, CCFP, FAAP, FCFP. "Does epidural analgesia increase rate of cesarean section?" *Can Fam Physician.* 2006 Apr 10; 52(4): 419–421.

96 Buckley, Sarah J. *Gentle Birth, Gentle Mothering: A Doctors Guide to Natural Childbirth and Gentle Early Parenting Choices.* Berkeley: Celestial Arts, 2009.

97 Childbirth Connection "VBAC Research and Evidence". http://www.childbirthconnection.org/giving-birth/vbac/research-evidence/.

98 Barrett JF, Hannah ME, Hutton EK, Willan AR, Allen AC, Armson BA, et al. "A randomized trial of planned cesarean or vaginal delivery for twin pregnancy." Twin Birth Study Collaborative Group. *N Engl J Med* 2013;369:1295–305; "Safe prevention of the primary cesarean delivery." Obstetric Care Consensus No. 1. American College of Obstetricians and Gynecologists. *Obstet Gynecol* 2014;123:693–711.

99 The International Weight Management in Pregnancy (i-WIP) Collaborative Group. "Effect of diet and physical activity based interventions in pregnancy on gestational weight gain and pregnancy outcomes: meta-analysis of individual participant data from randomised trials." The BMJ, 2017 doi: 10.1136/bmj.j3119.

100 "Approaches to limit interventions during labor and birth." ACOG Committee Opinion No. 766. American College of Obstetricians and Gynecologists. *Obstet Gynecol* 2019; 133:e164–73.

101 American College of Nurse-Midwives. "Intermittent auscultation for intrapartum fetal heart rate surveillance clinical bulletin no. 11." *J Midwifery Womens Health* 2010;55:397–403.

102 Rebecca L. Dekker, PhD, RN, APRN, 2012. "The Evidence on: Fetal Monitoring." Originally published on July 17, 2012 and updated on May 21, 2018, https://evidencebasedbirth.com/fetal-monitoring/.

103 "Intrapartum fetal heart rate monitoring: nomenclature, interpretation, and general management principles." ACOG Practice Bulletin No. 106. American College of Obstetricians and Gynecologists. *Obstet Gynecol* 2009;114:192–202.

104 American College of Obstetricians and Gynecologists. ACOG Practice Bulletin No. 106: "Intrapartum fetal heart rate monitoring: Nomenclature, interpretation, and general management principles." *Obstet Gynecol* 2009;114:192–202.

105 Waldman, Richard. "ACOG Practice Bulletin No. 198." *Obstetrics & Gynecology* 133, no. 1 (2019): 185. doi:10.1097/aog.0000000000003041; Cichowski S, Rogers R. Practice Bulletin No. 165: "Prevention and Management of Obstetric Lacerations at Vaginal Delivery." *Obstet Gynecol.* 2016 Jul;128(1):e1-e15. doi: 10.1097/AOG.0000000000001523.

106 Albers et al. 1996; Hastings-Tolsma et al. 2007; Mayerhofer et al. 2002; Murphy & Feinland 1998; Shorten, Donsante & Shorten 2002.

107 Hastings-Tolsma, M, Vincent, D, Emeis, C & Francisco, T 2007, "Getting through birth in one piece: protecting the perineum." *American Journal of Maternal Child Nursing*, vol. 32, no. 3, pp. 158–64; Dahlen, H, Ryan, M, Homer, CSE & Cooke, M 2007, "An Australian prospective cohort study of risk factors for severe perineal trauma during childbirth." *Midwifery*, vol. 23, pp. 196–203; Aasheim V, Nilsen A, Reinar L, Lukasse M. 2017. "Perineal techniques during the second stage of labour for reducing perineal trauma." Cochrane database of systematic reviews, June 2017. DOI 10.1002/14651858.cd006672.pub3.

108 Aasheim V, Nilsen A, Reinar L, Lukasse M. 2017. "Perineal techniques during the second stage of labour for reducing perineal trauma." Cochrane database of systematic reviews, June 2017. doi 10.1002/14651858.cd006672.pub3.

109 Nutter, E., Meyer, S., Shaw-Battista, J., et al. (2014a). "Waterbirth: an integrative analysis of peer-reviewed literature." *J Midwifery Womens Health* 59(3): 286–319.

110 Hong Jiang, Xu Qian, Guillermo Carroli, Paul Garner. 2017 "Selective versus routine use of episiotomy for vaginal birth." Cochrane database of systematic reviews, February 2017. doi: 10.1002/14651858.cd000081.pub3.

111 Hong Jiang, Xu Qian, Guillermo Carroli, Paul Garner. 2017 "Selective versus routine use of episiotomy for vaginal birth." Cochrane database of systematic reviews, February 2017. doi: 10.1002/14651858.cd000081.pub3.

112 Elseline Hoekzema, Erika Barba-Müller, Cristina Pozzobon, Marisol Picado, Florencio Lucco, David García-García, Juan Carlos Soliva, Adolf Tobeña, Manuel Desco, Eveline A Crone, Agustín Ballesteros, Susanna Carmona & Oscar Vilarroya. 2016. "Pregnancy leads to long-lasting changes in human brain structure." *Nature Neuroscience*. Volume 20, pages 287–296 (2017). https://doi.org/10.1038/nn.4458.

113 Pam Belluck, 2016. "Pregnancy Changes the Brain in Ways That May Help Mothering." *The New York Times*. Dec. 19, 2016. https://www.nytimes.com/2016/12/19/health/pregnancy-brain-change.html

114 Sanjeev Jain, MD, FAAP, 2018. "How Often and How Much Should Your Baby Eat?" American Academy of Pediatrics (Copyright © 2018) https://www.healthychildren.org/english/ages-stages/baby/feeding-nutrition/pages/how-often-and-how-much-should-your-baby-eat.aspx.

115 Caring for Your Baby and Young Child: Birth to Age 5, 6th Edition (Copyright © 2015 American Academy of Pediatrics) https://www.healthychildren.org/English/ages-stages/baby/formula-feeding/Pages/Amount-and-Schedule-of-Formula-Feedings.aspx.

116 Campbell-Yeo ML, Disher TC, Benoit BL, Johnston CC. "Understanding kangaroo care and its benefits to preterm infants." *Pediatric Health Med Ther*. 2015;6:15–32. Published 2015 Mar 18. doi:10.2147/PHMT.S51869.

117 Moore ER, Bergman N, Anderson GC, Medley N, 2016. "Early skin-to-skin contact for mothers and their healthy newborn infants." Cochrane Database Syst Rev. 2016 Nov 25;11:CD003519.

118 and 119 Moore, E. R., Bergman, N., Anderson, G. C., et al. (2016). Early skin-to-skin contact for mothers and their healthy newborn infants. Cochrane Database of Systematic Reviews, Issue 11. Art. No.: CD003519.

120 American Academy of Pediatrics Supports Childhood Sleep Guidelines, 2016. Last updated June 13, 2016. https://www.aap.org/en-us/about-the-aap/aap-press-room/Pages/American-Academy-of-Pediatrics-Supports-Childhood-Sleep-Guidelines.aspx.

121 Kiel EJ, Hummel AC, Luebbe AM. "Cortisol secretion and change in sleep problems in early childhood: Moderation by maternal overcontrol." *Biol Psychol*. 2015;107:52–60. doi:10.1016/j.biopsycho.2015.03.001.

122 Brazelton, T.B. "Crying in infancy." *Pediatrics* 1962; 29(4):579–588.

123 Ko, J.Y., Rockhill, K.M., Tong, V.T., Morrow, B., Farr, S.L. (2017). "Trends in Postpartum Depressive Symptoms—27 States," 2004, 2008, and 2012 (link is external). MMWR Morb Mortal Wkly Rep; 66: 153–158.

124 Poyatos-León, R, García-Hermoso, A, Sanabria-Martínez, G, Álvarez-Bueno, C, Cavero-Redondo, I, Martínez-Vizcaíno, V. "Effects of exercise-based interventions on postpartum depression: A meta-analysis of randomized controlled trials." *Birth*. 2017; 44: 200–208. https://doi.org/10.1111/birt.12294.

125 Hughes H., 2008. "Management of postpartum loss of libido." *J Fam Health Care*. 2008;18(4):123-5.

126 Sharon Lerner, 2015. "The real war on families". In These Times. August 18, 2015. http://inthesetimes.com/article/18151/the-real-war-on-families.

127 US Department of Labor, 1993. Family and Medical Leave Act. https://www.dol.gov/whd/fmla/.

128 http://www.nationalpartnership.org/our-work/workplace/paid-leave-resources.html.

129 Raipuria, Harinder Dosanjh, Briana Lovett, Laura Lucas, and Victoria Hughes. "A Literature Review of Midwifery-Led Care in Reducing Labor and Birth Interventions." *Nursing for Womens Health* 22, no. 5 (2018): 387-400. doi:10.1016/j.nwh.2018.07.002.

130 Lauren Slate, 2002. *Love Works Like This: Moving from One Kind of Life to Another*. Random House; First Edition edition (May 14, 2002).

131 Brewer, Sarah Dr. *The Pregnant Body Book*. New York: DK Publishing, 2011.

132 Segal, Scott, MD, MHCM, 2010. "Labor Epidural Analgesia and Maternal Fever" *Anesthesia & Analgesia* December 2010 Volume 111 Issue 6 p 1467–1475. doi: 10.1213/ANE.0b013e3181f713d4.

133 American Optometric Association. "Infant Vision: Birth to 24 Months of Age." https://www.aoa.org/patients-and-public/good-vision-throughout-life/childrens-vision/infant-vision-birth-to-24-months-of-age.

134 American Academy of Dermatology. "Is that acne on my baby's face?" https://www.aad.org/public/diseases/acne-and-rosacea/newborn-acne; Eichenfield LF, Krakowski AC, et al. "Evidence-based recommendations for the diagnosis and treatment of pediatric acne." *Pediatrics*. 2013;131 Suppl 3:S163-86.

135 Huber A, 1976. "The frequency of physiologic vaginal bleeding of newborn infants." *Zentralbl Gynakol.* 1976;98(16):1017-20.

Index